KAMA SUTRA
OF
SEXUAL POSITIONS

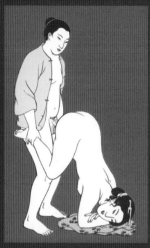
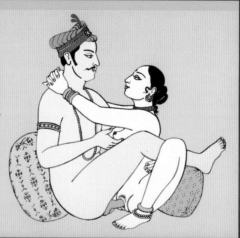
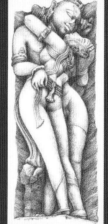
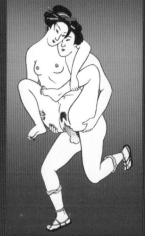

THE TANTRIC ART OF LOVE
Sensual Practices from *Secret Sexual Positions*

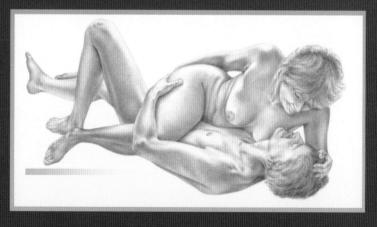

Kenneth Ray Stubbs, Ph.D.
Illustrated by Kyle Spencer and Richard Stodart

Jeremy P. Tarcher/Putnam

a member of Penguin Putnam Inc.

New York

While the author has made every effort to provide accurate telephone numbers and Internet addresses at the time of publication, neither the publisher nor the author assumes any responsibility for errors, or for changes that occur after publication.

Most Tarcher/Putnam books are available at special quantity discounts for bulk purchase for sales promotions, premiums, fund-raising, and educational needs. Special books or book excerpts also can be created to fit specific needs. For details, write Putnam Special Markets, 375 Hudson Street, New York, NY 10014.

A Word of Caution

The purpose of this book is to educate. It is not intended to give medical or psychological therapy. Whenever there is concern about physical or emotional illness, a qualified professional should be consulted. Not all the sexual positions in this book are for every body. Some of the positions were accomplished only after years of yogic practice.
The author, illustrator, and publisher shall have neither liability nor responsibility to any person or entity with respect to any loss, damage, injury, or ailment caused or alleged to be caused directly or indirectly by the information or lack of information in this book.

Jeremy P. Tarcher/Putnam
a member of
Penguin Putnam Inc.
375 Hudson Street
New York, NY 10014
www.penguinputnam.com

The exercises in this book have been previously published in
Secret Sexual Positions © 1998 Kenneth Ray Stubbs, Ph.D.

First published in 2001 by Secret Garden Publishing

First Jeremy P. Tarcher/Putnam Edition 2003

Library of Congress Cataloging-in-Publication Data

Stubbs, Kenneth Ray.
Kama Sutra of sexual positions : the tantric art of love / by Kenneth Ray Stubbs ;
illustrated by Kyle Spencer and Richard Stodart.
p.   cm.
Originally published: Tucson, Az. : Secret Garden Publishers, 2001.
ISBN 1-58542-218-5
1. Våtsyåyana. Kåmasåtra.   2. Sex instruction.   3. Love.   4. Sexual excitement.
I. Spencer, Kyle.   II. Stodart, Richard.   III. Title.
HQ31.S9895   2003   2002032030
613.9'07—dc21

Printed in Korea

1   3   5   7   9   10   8   6   4   2

This book is printed on acid-free paper. ∞

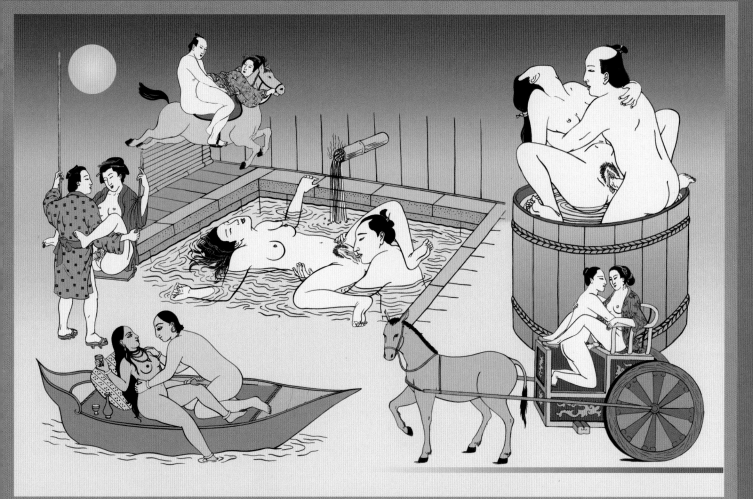

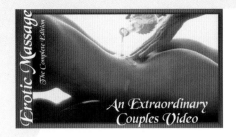

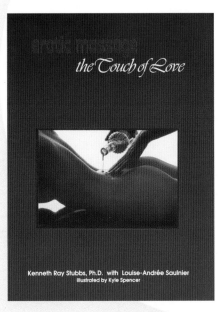

Also by the same author

Erotic Massage: The Tantric Touch of Love

The Essential Tantra: A Modern Guide to Sacred Sexuality

Secret Sexual Positions: Ancient Techniques for Modern Lovers

Erotic Passions: A Guide to Orgasmic Massage, Sensual Bathing, Oral Pleasuring, and Ancient Sexual Positions

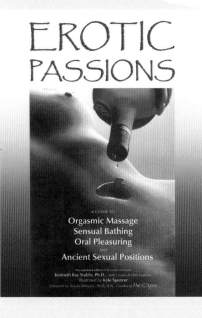

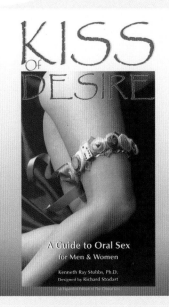

Contents

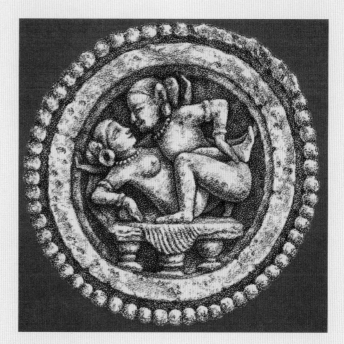

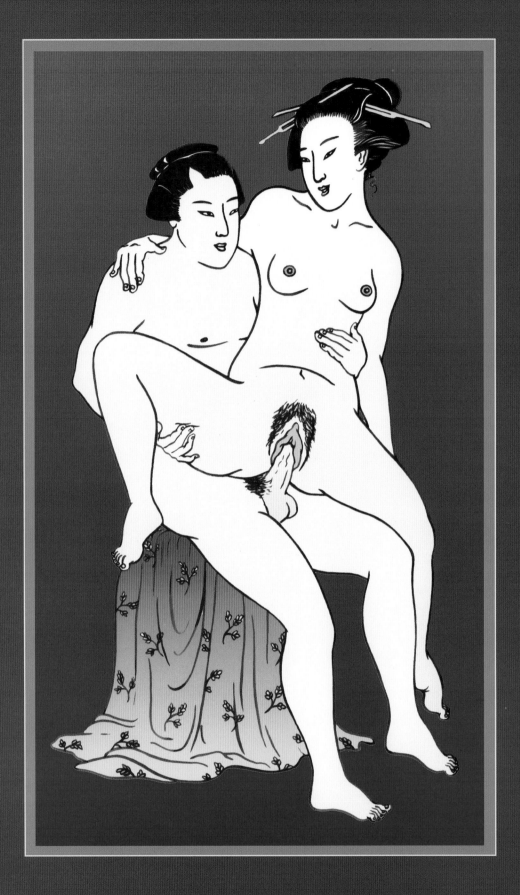

Introduction

From thirteenth-century India on the temple walls of Konarak, we easily see life-size stone carvings revealing women and men in almost every conceivable sexual embrace.

In the *Ishimpo* (ee shem' poh), a thousand-year-old Japanese medical text, we are instructed in a healing sexual position named the Wild Horse Leaps, where the female's feet are lifted toward the heavens and the "jade stalk" is inserted deeply into the "jade gate."

From the biblical Song of Songs, we glean a hint of the pleasures of oral-vaginal sex—a thousand years before Christianity: "I am my beloved's, and my beloved is mine: he feedeth among the lilies."[1]

From the early sixteenth-century North African Arabic world, we read *The Perfumed Garden*: "Let praise be given to God that He has created woman with her beauty and appetizing flesh: that He has endowed her with hair, waist, and throat, breasts that swell, and amorous gestures which increase desire.[2] . . . God has granted us the kiss on the mouth, the cheeks and the mouth, as also the sucking of luscious lips, to provoke an erection at a favorable time."[3]

To many other peoples of many other times, the intertwining of sin and sex would appear strange, perhaps incomprehensible. To pronounce sex as forbidden fruit might even be heresy.

Sex is primordial. Sexual energy is sacred. Sexual pleasure is healing and transformative. These conceptions were inherent in the worldview of many ancients who tasted of the tree of knowledge and learned that the fruit should never be forbidden.

The original Kama Sutra was written by a holy man in India almost two millennia ago. Today in the West, "Kama Sutra" has often come to be interpreted as a bible of sex. It is in this sense that I chose the title *Kama Sutra of Sexual Positions* as an introduction to ancient lovers of many different cultures where the sexual and the sacred were the weaver of the tapestry of life.

Most of the images herein are based on paintings or written descriptions from India, China, and Japan. Some of the methods go back to very early writings. Some come to us from the probably mythical Chinese Yellow Emperor and his three wise-woman sexual mentors of some 5,000 years ago. In all likelihood, most of the sexual methods here antedate recorded history, for our sexuality is inherent.

While much of the available ancient lover material often assumes a male reader and a male acting as the directing partner, the underlying tone is usually far more egalitarian, sensual, and empathetic than much of the sexually explicit material generated in the West in recent centuries.

A complete set of sexual positions is far from the goal here. This is a fun book to use in contemplating possibilities from ancient lovers, human beings who came before us and who sought and discovered the sweet beauty of the fruit.

The Illustrations

Some of the illustrations are based on photographs of modern lovers interpreting the writings and paintings from ancient lovers. Several of the people in these images are quite accomplished in yoga, as can be seen in the flexibility required in some of the positions. Most of the lovers are experienced in different forms of meditation, as seen.in their eye connections.

The largest set of illustrations presents a wide variety of positions by ancient lovers. These are intended to simply convey the sexual embrace itself with a hint of the garments, accessories, and environment of some ancient cultures.

Another set of illustrations comes from sensual sculptures on temple walls in India. While an embarrassment to some contemporary puritanical Indians, these sculptures are among the finest erotic art in the world.

Finally, the classic Japanese erotic art style known as *shunga* gives us a refreshingly different view of sexual embrace.

While coming to us mostly from writings and art over many centuries and many cultural milieus, all the illustrations here are by Kyle Spencer. Often the positions included are the result of my instruction to her to have fun with this project of 100 illustrations. I suggested she vary patterns in garments, envision new settings, and basically follow her artistic heart.

Kama Sutra of Sexual Positions is a revised, all-color edition of my earlier *Secret Sexual Positions*. I invited Richard Stodart, another artist, to bring color to the original black-and-white illustrations and to compose some of them as montages. I encouraged him to express his artistic vision to celebrate the dynamic diversities of the sexual embrace.

The Text

We are greatly indebted to Sir Richard Burton (1821–1890) for translating into English three very important erotological texts from non-Western cultures. The famous Kama Sutra comes from India, compiled by Vatsyayana about the fourth century C.E. However, that book is based on earlier writings, possibly from the third century B.C.E., with an earlier source work dating back to about the eighth century B.C.E. (Note that B.C.E. means *Before Common Era* and is equivalent to B.C. Similarly, C.E. is equivalent to A.D.)

Derived from the Kama Sutra, the *Ananga-Ranga* by Kalyana Malla comes from thirteenth-century C.E. India after Islamic influences. The third of Burton's translations, *The Perfumed Garden* by Sheikh Nefzawi, is from the Islamic culture of early sixteenth-century North African Arabic Tunis.

Going farther east, we have the Japanese *Ishimpo,* compiled in the late tenth century C.E. and based on Chinese medical texts and teachings going back to the probably mythical Chinese Yellow Emperor, possibly around 2700 B.C.E.

Kama Sutra of Sexual Positions adapts and summarizes some of the sexual positions recommended by these ancient cultures. References to animals are common, and the missionary position is but one possibility.

The poetry accompanying some of the images is my interpretation and expression of writings from poets and mystics through the ages. *Lover, nature,* and *God/Goddess* are often a spiraling oneness for these mystics, who commonly danced in the realm of the sacred and the sexual. At times, my words might be only a distant resemblance of the ancient poet's voice as I speak through my modern consciousness.

The biblical Song of Songs, often attributed to Solomon, is the basis for most of the poems. Inanna is the Sumarian Goddess Queen of Heaven and Earth. Her legend predates Solomon's rule by at least two millennia, and the biblical Abraham was born in this ancient land of Sumer.

Rumi, born in Afghanistan in the thirteenth century C.E., was a conventional teacher until at thirty-seven he met a wandering Islamic mystic. Lalla, in fourteenth-century Kashmir, left her home at twenty-four and became a wandering mystic, sometimes dancing naked in the streets in ecstasy. Longchenpa was a fourteenth-century Tibetan master in the Tantric tradition. St. Teresa of Avila was a sixteenth-century Spanish Catholic nun who became known for her overtly ecstatic expressions as she communed with God. Finally, Chaco is now a set of ruins located in the southwestern U.S. These were sacred ceremonial structures built by a highly evolved Native American culture beginning in the mid-ninth century to mark the yearly cycle of the sun and the eighteen-and-a-half-year cycle of the moon.

Conclusion

The following images and words can serve as inspiration for those of us raised in a consciousness were sex is forbidden fruit. Even if the fruit is not forbidden for us, there is always more to learn, more pleasure to share. My suggestion to the reader is to explore the diversities. Have fun. Open the imagination. Sip the nectar and eat "of the fruit of the tree which is in the midst of the garden."[4]

In the embrace, become One.

---

[1] Song of Songs 6:3.

[2] Sir Richard Burton, trans., Charles Fowkes, ed., *The Perfumed Garden* (Rochester, VT: Park Street Press, 1992), p. 11.

[3] Ibid., p. 10.

[4] Genesis 3:3.

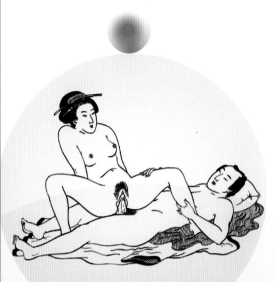

*S*outh winds,
north winds
I call to you
My fruit has ripened
on the vine

Come, breathe upon
my garden
so my lover might find
his way
in the night

inspired by
the Song of Songs

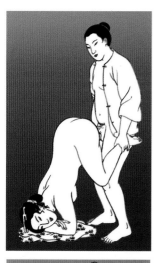

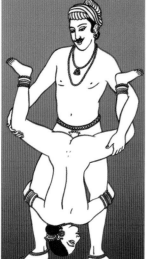

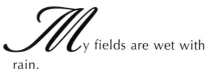y fields are wet with rain.
Who will plow my fertile earth?

My blossoms awaken in the morning.
        Who will breathe my fragrance into his flute so I might dance on the wind?

My moon is full.
My figs and grapes are swollen.
        Who will feast in my temple?

*inspired by
the legends of Inanna*

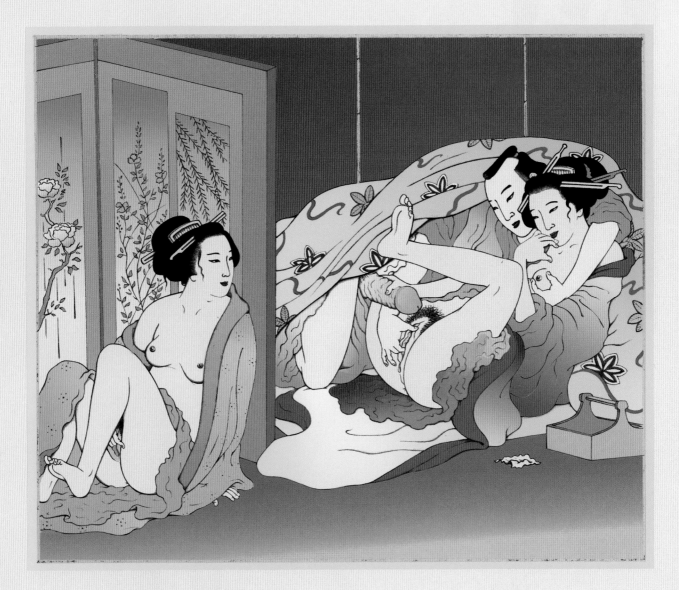

Ancient Lovers

She went to the sheepfold, to the shepherd. . . .

When she leaned back against the apple tree, her vulva was wondrous to behold.

Rejoicing at her wondrous vulva, . . . Inanna applauded herself. . . .

As for me, Inanna,

Who will plow my vulva?

Who will plow my high field?

Who will plow my wet ground?

Who will station the ox there?

Her lover, Dumuzi the King, replies he will.

Then plow my vulva, man of my heart!

Plow my vulva![1]

This story of Inanna comes from some of humankind's earliest known writings. Almost 4,000-year-old cuneiform tablets depict Inanna (ee nah' nuh), the goddess, Queen of Heaven and Earth, as revering her vulva, its beauty, and her sexual desires. Her religious legend, which may go back more than 5,500 years, is from Sumer, a small part of the land area we now generally call the Middle East.

The entangled web of our modern sexual consciousness to a great extent also comes from Sumer, though mostly from a very different religious lineage than Inanna's. About 4,000 years ago, Abraham, strictly obeying what he believed to be the commands of his god Yahweh, left Ur, once the capital city of Sumer, to find a new land which his "seed" would inherit.

Abraham is the patriarchal progenitor of Judaism, Christianity, and Islam. The religious beliefs and societal laws that have sprung forth from these three pervasive legacies provide the foundation of many of the modern lovers' sexual beliefs and customs.

The male gender decides; the female gender follows. Not only are the spirit and the body different; the spirit is morally superior. Pleasures of the flesh are sinful. Sex is solely for procreation. Only the missionary position is condoned. The wages of sin are illness and death.

While many of us modern lovers would contend that most or all of these beliefs are old-fashioned, such tenants remain deeply embedded in our collective unconscious. (Even at the end of the twentieth century, the Chief Justice of the U.S. Supreme Court wrote, "Public nudity is the *evil* the state seeks to prevent. . . ."[2] [italics added].)

In contrast, also in the entangled web of our modern sexual consciousness, a compelling anomaly exists among the Jewish and Christian canonical texts. A thousand years after Abraham, Solomon inherited the throne from David to become the most extolled king of Israel. With a probably exaggerated estimate of 700 wives and 300 concubines, Solomon no doubt had ample opportunity to explore the amatory realms. Often though probably inaccurately attributed to him, the Song of Songs graces our minds with images lovers would feel:

> *Let him kiss me with the kisses of his mouth: for thy love is better than wine.* [Song of Songs 1:2]

> *A bundle of myrrh is my well-beloved unto me; he shall lie all night betwixt my breasts.* [Song of Songs 1:13]

> *I am my beloved's, and his desire is toward me.* [Song of Songs 7:10]

These poetic praises from the Song of Songs, or Song of Solomon, often bear striking resemblances to Inanna's hymns. This should come as no surprise. Solomon built temples for a variety of female and male deities other than Yahweh, and the Sumerian civilization was part of his roots.

Solomon's kingdom was a bustling empire of commerce and far-reaching alliances bringing cultural contact with those far beyond a provincial world of sheepherders and purist priests. Goddess traditions honoring the cycles of the moon as well as earth-centered fertility ceremonies celebrating the fecundity of plants, herds, and humans alike abounded both within the diverse early Hebrew people and in surrounding cultures.

Nonetheless, a priesthood with a single, wrathful, male deity was to be the dominating power for the early Hebrews. Even ethnic cleansing of other male and female deities' followers, including the slaughter of all men, women, and children, was not uncommon.[3] Sometimes, though, the gold, domesticated animals, and female virgins were spared and made property.[4]

The Christianity of Paul (d. 62–68 C.E.) followed, then the conversion of the Roman Empire to Christian doctrine (early 4th century), later the sex-is-sin philosophies of Augustine (345–430) and Aquinas (1225–1274). Eventually, either with active promotion or acquiescence from the Church of Rome or Protestant powers, over 500 years of formal Inquisitions were to leave little semblance of spiritual traditions espousing sex as a sacrament. After perhaps up to nine million burnings at the stake and other tortured deaths,[5] European Christenom had basically committed genocide on those who would dare to engage in spiritual practices which Inanna, Astarte, Aphrodite, and other Western European sex-embracing deities might proclaim.

In the Americas, Balboa would unleash his large, specially trained attack dogs on indigenous peoples for their common sexual customs deemed heretical to the Church of Rome. Add the influence of the puritanical wings of the Protestants, and we find the Western twentieth-century modern lover inheriting the legacy of a virtual sexual wasteland.

For almost 4,000 years, our principal cultural heritage has known and taught little in the arts of love and sex. Moreover, a wondrous unity of sex and spirit has been philosophically unconscionable.

❦

And then there was Sir Richard Francis Burton.

Burton (1821–1890) was a famous British explorer and prolific author, with forty-three volumes on his explorations and almost thirty volumes of translations.

Based on his fluency in forty languages and dialects as well as extensive experiences of "going native" in India and in Muslim cultures, Burton translated and secretly printed the Kama Sutra in 1883, the *Ananga-Ranga* in 1885, and *The Perfumed Garden* in 1886. (Often co-translating with Burton was his close friend Foster Arbuthnot.)

Risking prosecution, imprisonment, and disgrace in Victorian Britain, Burton was a bicultural messenger, clandestinely bringing glimpses of ancient lovers' arts of love and sex long suppressed in the West. Probably more than any other single individual in the English language, Burton lifted the sex-is-sin veil so that we might see a far healthier possibility of our sexual selves.

Kama is the god of love in India. Similar to Cupid, Kama has a bow that shoots love-producing flower arrows. The term *kama* itself can be translated as "love, pleasure, sensual gratification."

A sutra is a collection of concise statements, written so that they might be more easily memorized. In the case of the Kama Sutra, scripturelike advice provides guidance not only on succeeding in the arts of love and sex, for which the book is most known, but also on attaining virtue and wealth. Ironically, with sexual censorship waning in the 1960s and various printings of this formerly illicit treasure becoming commonly available, it is the sections on virtue and wealth that are often conveniently edited out.

Writing the Kama Sutra somewhere between the fourth century B.C.E. and the fourth century C.E., Vatsyayana described himself in the conclusion of this significant compilation and adaptation of previous writings in India:

> The Kama Sutra was composed, according to the precepts of Holy Writ, for the benefit of the world, by Vatsyayana, while leading the life of a religious student, and wholly engaged in the contemplation of the Deity.[6]

Where sexual union can symbolize the union of cosmic energies, it would not seem strange that a holy person could write a text describing the arts of love and sex. Harmony in the universe and harmony between lovers are but a mirror of each other.

Beginning in the third and forth centuries in India, a dynamic spiritual movement known

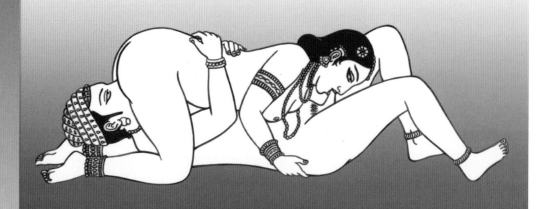

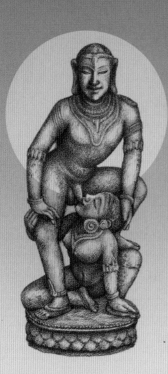

*T*he shade of
your apricot tree
comforts me from
the midday sun

The redness of the
pomegranate seed
the nectar of the grape
slip from your lips
to mine

Your lily's fragrance
lifts me to a realm
where midday and
midnight are one

I am lost in your
garden

*inspired by
the Song of Songs*

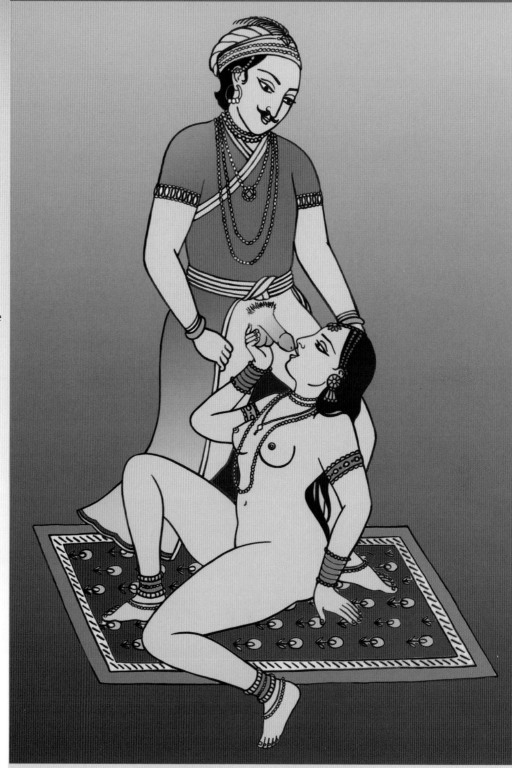

as Tantra (tahn' tra) began to appear. By that time many of the dominant religious themes emphasized asceticism: Only by denying the body and abstaining from pleasure could one lead a holy life. Suffering and penance, including self-inflicted pain, were next to godliness.

Tantra, to an ascetic, might be considered hedonistic indulgence. For a Tantric adept, all of life and death is embraced. Every experience, especially sex, is an opportunity to discover more deeply our inherent nature.

Various meditations, including sexual ceremonies and positions, some apparently adapted from the Kama Sutra information, were developed to teach the follower on this path. Through meditation, our experience of daily existence—the good, the bad, the ugly, the beautiful—is transformed from attachment to enlightenment.

Tantra, indeed, is a path, often requiring many years of commitment to various meditations, or "surrender to," as a Tantrika might conceptualize it. This path is for those seeking more than a new romantic or sexual skill. Nonetheless, this diverse philosophy, which has had significant influences on Hinduism and Buddhism, gives us some insight into the ancient lovers' embrace of the sacred and the sexual, a view far outside the sex-is-sin perversion pervading our Western sexual legacy.

In late twelfth-century India, the *Ananga-Ranga*, or *The Hindu Art of Love*, was written by Kalyana Malla. Arriving after Islamic conquerings and cultural influences, this book, however, is derived from the Kama Sutra. Emphasizing a marriage relationship, the manual accentuates the mutual pleasure and harmony of the genders:

> And thus all you who read this
> book shall know how delicious
> an instrument is woman, when
> artfully played upon; how capable she is of producing the
> most exquisite harmony; of executing the most complicated
> variations and of giving the
> divinest pleasures.[7]

The third of Burton's translations, *The Perfumed Garden* by Sheikh Nefzawi, comes to us from the Islamic culture of early sixteenth-century North African Arabic Tunis. Here again, pleasure more than procreation is praised:

> If you wish to experience an
> agreeable copulation, one that
> gives equal satisfaction and pleasure to both parties, it is necessary to frolic with the woman and
> excite her with nibbling, kissing,
> and caressing. Turn her over on
> the bed, sometimes on her back,
> sometimes on her belly, until you
> see by her eyes that the moment
> of pleasure has arrived. . . .[8]

No slam-bam-thank-ya-ma'am aura is exalted in these treatises translated by Burton, except, of course, when such encounters are mutually rewarding for both partners.

Looking to the ancient lovers farther east in China and Japan, we often find more of a medical emphasis in the numerous sexual texts, such as the twenty-eighth section of the Japanese *Ishimpo*. This is a compilation and adaptation of many earlier Chinese texts often extensively influenced by Taoist spiritual philosophy. (*Tao* is pronounced *dow*, like *wow* beginning with a *d*.)

> One gets longevity by loving the
> essence, cultivating the spiritual,
> and partaking of many kinds of
> medicines; if you do not know
> the ways of intercourse, partaking of herbs is of no benefit.[9]

Being in harmony with our inner nature might be considered the quintessence of Taoist philosophy, dating back to at least the fourth century B.C.E. in China. Sexual health is an essential aspect of health if we are to live in balance with Heaven and Earth. So part of a physician's role would be to facilitate our sexuality remaining in harmony with the other aspects of our life—including knowing which sexual positions help heal which conditions.

Also striking to the Western modern lover's ear is the sensual ambiance of the poetic language describing sex. "The clouds and the rain" and "the mists and the rain" refer to intercourse. A penis is a "jade stalk" or a "bamboo horse." A "pearl on the jade step" is a clitoris, while a "coral gate," "jade pavilion," and "magic field" are the female genitals in general. "Fire inside the jade pavilion" would be a woman's orgasm.

❧

Sexuality as sacrament or as forbidden fruit—both themes are apparent as we examine our human history. Kama Sutra and other ancient texts give us a hint of the world of ancient lovers who danced in the center of the sacred circle.

Kama Sutra of Sexual Positions is my interpretation and my honoring of the teachings of these ancient lovers.

> *When we dance naked*
> *I hear your heartbeat*
> *There I soar*
> > *in the spiral*
> *There I embrace*
> > *the circle*

> *Is this why*
> *God gave us lovers?*

[1] Diane Wolkstein and Samuel Noah Kramer, *Inanna: Queen of Heaven and Earth* (New York: Harper & Row, 1983), various selections.

[2] "Ban on Nude Dancing Backed by High Court," *Los Angeles Times*, Home Ed., 22 June 1991, pt. A, p. A-1.

[3] "So the LORD our God delivered into our hands Og also, the king of Bashan, and all his people . . . and we took all his cities at that time . . . threescore cities . . . utterly destroying the men, women, and children, of every city." [Deuteronomy 3:3–6]

[4] "And the booty, being the rest of the prey which the men of war had caught, was six hundred thousand and seventy thousand and five thousand sheep, and threescore and twelve thousand beeves, and threescore and one thousand asses, and thirty and two thousand persons in all, of women that had not known man by lying with him." [Numbers 31:32–35]

(See *When God Was a Woman* by Merlin Stone [New York: Harvest/Harcourt Brace Jovanovich, 1976] for an extensive discussion of the early Hebrews and the surrounding sex-positive cultures.)

[5] See Elinor W. Gadon, *The Once and Future Goddess* (New York: HarperCollins, 1989), p. 113, and Starhawk, *Dreaming the Dark*, new edition (Boston: Beacon Press, 1982, 1988), p. 187.

[6] Sir Richard Burton and F. F. Arbuthnot, trans., Charles Fowkes, ed., *The Illustrated Kama Sutra, Ananga-Ranga, Perfumed Garden* (Rochester, VT: Park Street Press, 1991), p. 18.

[7] Ibid., p. 68.

[8] Sir Richard Burton, trans., Charles Fowkes, ed., *The Perfumed Garden* (Rochester, VT: Park Street Press, 1992), p. 32.

[9] Howard S. Levy and Akira Ishihara, trans., *The Tao of Sex* (Lower Lake, CA: Integral Publishing, 1989), p. 17.

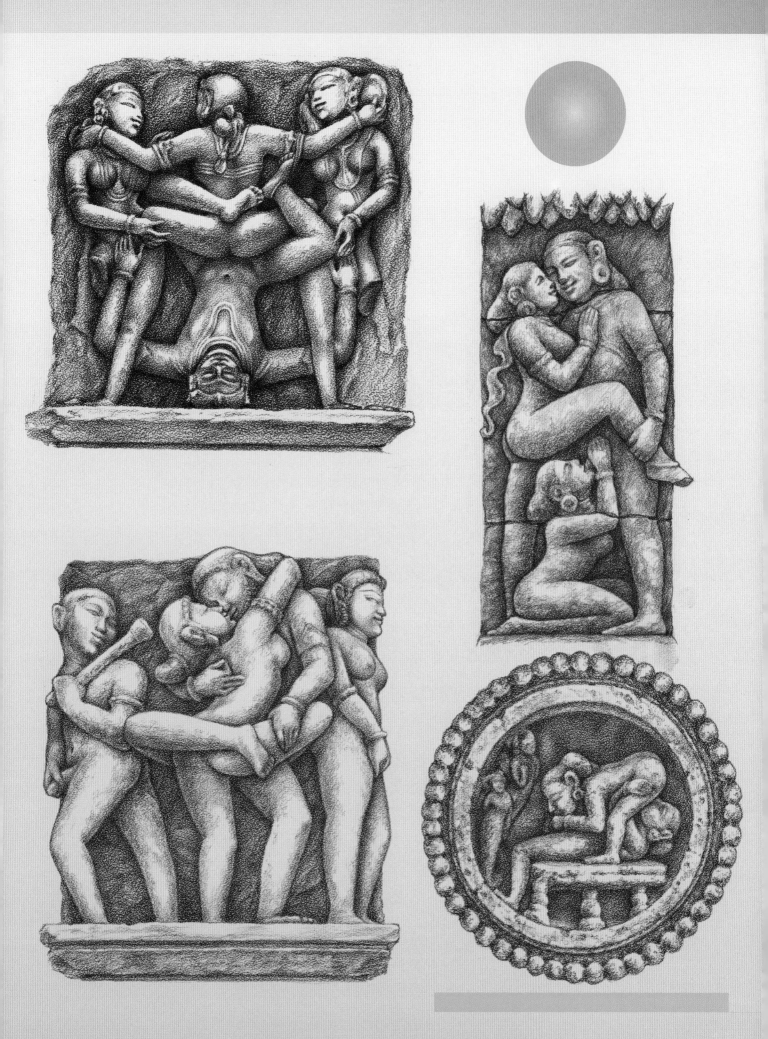

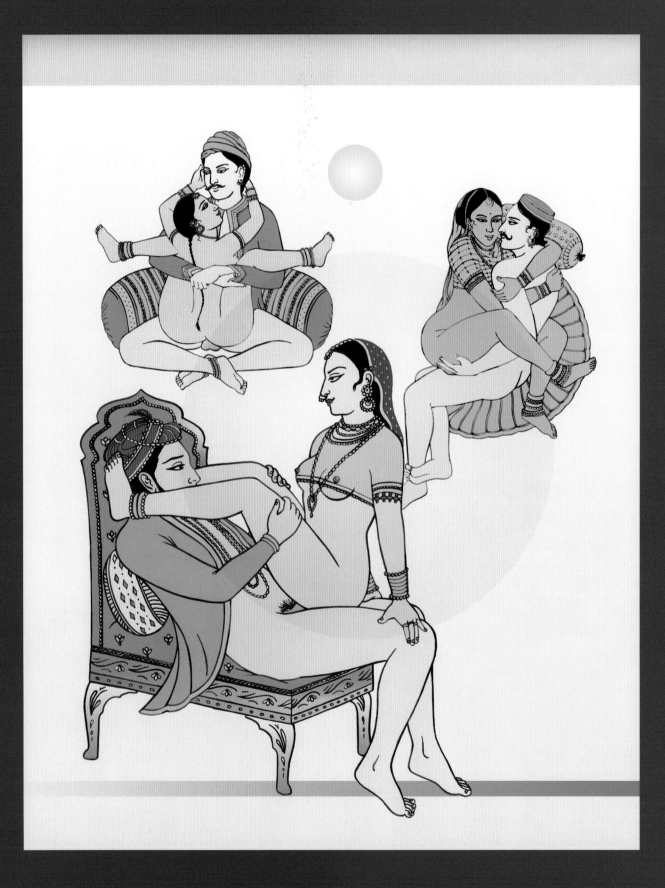

Kama Sutra

by
Vatsyayana

Selected and Adapted Positions

Most descriptions in Sir Richard Burton's translation indicating the male being in charge of all the actions are edited so that the female is now more of an equal participant and initiator.

An ingenious person should multiply the kinds of congress after the fashion of the different kinds of beasts and of birds. For these different kinds of congress, performed according to the . . . liking of each individual, generate love, friendship, and respect in the hearts of women.

Widely opened position
When she lowers her head and raises her middle parts.

Yawning position
When she raises her thighs and keeps them wide apart.

Position of Indrani
When she places her thighs with her legs doubled on them upon her sides.

Clasping position
When the legs of both the male and the female are stretched straight out over each other. It is of two kinds, the side position and the supine position.

Pressing position
When, after congress has begun in the clasping position, the woman presses her lover with her thighs.

Twining position
When the woman places one of her thighs across the thigh of her lover.

Mare's position
When a woman forcibly holds in her yoni [female genitalia] the lingam [penis] after it is in.

Rising position
When the female raises both of her thighs straight up.

Yawning position
When she raises both of her legs, and places them on her lover's shoulder.

Pressed position

When the legs are contracted, and thus held by the lover before his bosom.

Half-pressed position

When only one of her legs is stretched out.

Splitting of a bamboo position

When the woman places one of her legs on her lover's shoulder, and stretches the other out, and then places the latter on his shoulder, and stretches out the other, and continues to do so alternately.

Fixing of a nail

When one of her legs is placed on the head, and the other is stretched out.

Crab's position

When both the legs of the woman are contracted and placed on her stomach.

Packed position

When the thighs are raised and placed one upon the other.

Lotuslike position

When the shanks are placed one upon the other.

Turning position

When a man, during congress, turns round, and enjoys the woman without leaving her, while she embraces him round the back all the time.

Supported congress

When a man and a woman support themselves on each other's bodies, or on a wall, or pillar, and thus while standing.

Suspended congress

When a man supports himself against a wall, and the woman, sitting on his hands joined together and held underneath her, throws her arms round his neck, and putting her thighs alongside his waist, moves herself by her feet, which are touching the wall against which the man is leaning.

Congress of a cow

When a woman stands on her hands and feet like a quadruped, and her lover mounts her like a bull. At this time everything that is ordinarily done on the bosom should be done on the back.

United congress

When a man enjoys two women at the same time, both of whom love him equally.

Lower congress

When congress is in the anus.

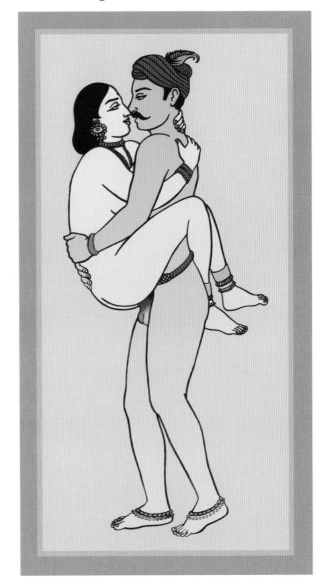

*S*hould you find
my beloved
tending his flock
in the hills,
lean closely
to his ear
and beckon him
run as the gazelle
to my lips
for I am faint
with the fever
of love.

inspired by
the Song of Songs

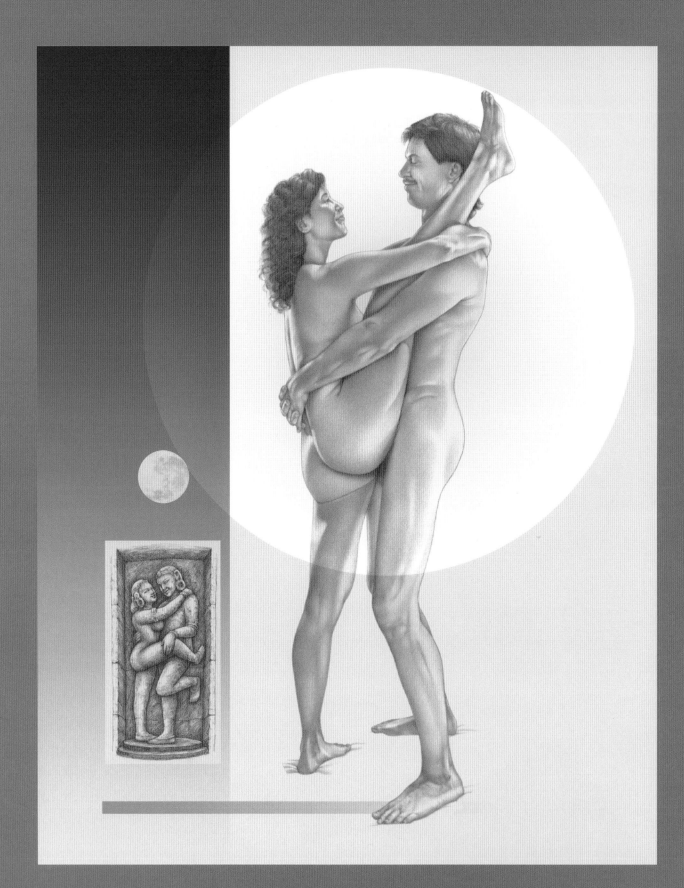

The Perfumed Garden

by
Sheikh Nefzawi

Selected and Adapted Positions

Most descriptions in Sir Richard Burton's translation indicating the male being in charge of all the actions are edited so that the female is now more of an equal participant and initiator. Brackets indicate a significant modification of content or terms.

First posture

The woman lies on her back and raises her thighs; then, getting between her legs, the man introduces his member. Gripping the ground with his toes, he will be able to move in a suitable manner. This posture is a good one for males who have long members.

Second posture

If the male's member is short, the woman lies on her back and he raises her legs in the air so that her toes touch her ears. Her buttocks being thus raised, the vulva is thrown forward. Now he introduces his member.

Third posture

She lies on the ground and he gets between her thighs; then, with one of her legs on his shoulder and the other under his arm, he penetrates her.

Fourth posture

She stretches on the ground and puts her legs on his shoulders; in that position his member will be exactly opposite her vulva which will be lifted off the ground. That is the moment he introduces his member.

Fifth posture

The woman lies on her side on the ground; then, lying down and getting between her thighs, the man introduces his member. This posture is apt to give rise to rheumatic or sciatic pains.

Sixth posture

The woman rests on her knees and elbows in the position for prayer. In this posture the vulva stands out behind. He enters her thus.

Seventh posture

The woman is on her side; then the male, sitting on his heels, will place her top leg on his nearest shoulder and her other leg against his thighs. She will keep on her side, and he will be between her legs. He introduces his member and moves her backward and forward with his hands.

Eighth posture

With the woman on her back, he kneels astride her.

Ninth posture

The woman rests, either face forward or the reverse, against a slightly raised platform, her feet remaining on the ground and her body projecting in front. She will thus present her vulva to the man's member, which he will introduce.

Tenth posture

The woman is on a rather low divan, grasping the woodwork with her hands; then with her legs on his hips and gripping his body, he will introduce his member, at the same time grasping the divan. When the lovers begin to work, they let their movements keep time.

Eleventh posture

The woman lies on her back with her buttocks raised by a cushion placed under them. She puts the soles of her feet together with the man between her thighs.

The closure

The woman lies on her back, her buttocks raised with a cushion; then the man gets between her legs, keeping his toes on the floor, and presses her thighs against her chest. Now he passes his hands under her arms to clasp her to himself, or tightly grips her shoulders. That done, he introduces his member and draws her towards himself at the moment of ejaculation. This posture may be painful for the woman, for, with her thighs pressed on her chest and her buttocks raised with the cushion, the walls of the vagina are forced together, and, as a consequence—the uterus being pushed forward—there is not enough room for the penis, which can only be inserted with difficulty, and which impinges on the womb. This posture should only be used when the penis is short and soft.

The frog's posture

The woman is on her back and her thighs raised till her heels are close to her buttocks. Now the man seats himself in front of her vulva and introduces his member; then putting her knees under his armpits and, grasping the upper part of her arms, he draws her to himself at the propitious moment.

The clasping of hands and feet

With the woman on her back, the man sits on his heels between her thighs and grips the floor with his toes; she will now put her legs round his body and he will put his arms about her neck.

The raised legs posture

While the woman is lying on her back, the man takes hold of her legs and, holding them close together, raises them until her soles point to the ceiling; then clasping her between his thighs, he introduces his member, taking care at the same time not to let her legs fall.

The goat's posture

The woman lies on her side and stretches out the bottom leg. The man crouches down between her thighs, lifts her top leg and introduces his member. He holds her by the arms or shoulders.

The Archimedean screw

While the man is lying on his back, the woman sits on his member, keeping her face towards his. She then places her hands on the bed, at the same time keeping her belly off his; she now moves up and down and, if the man is light in weight, he may move as well. If the woman wishes to kiss the man, she need only lay her arms on the bed.

The ancient swing

The woman is suspended face upwards from the ceiling by means of four cords [wide sashes] attached to her hands and feet and another supporting the middle of her body.

The spiral between
the heavens
and the earth
The circle between
the nights
and the days
circling into seasons

When we dance naked
I hear your heartbeat
There I soar
in the spiral
There I embrace
the circle

Is this why
God gave us lovers?

inspired by
Lalla

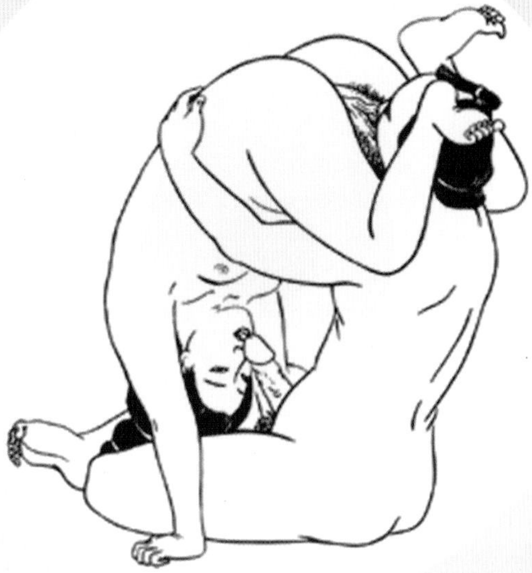

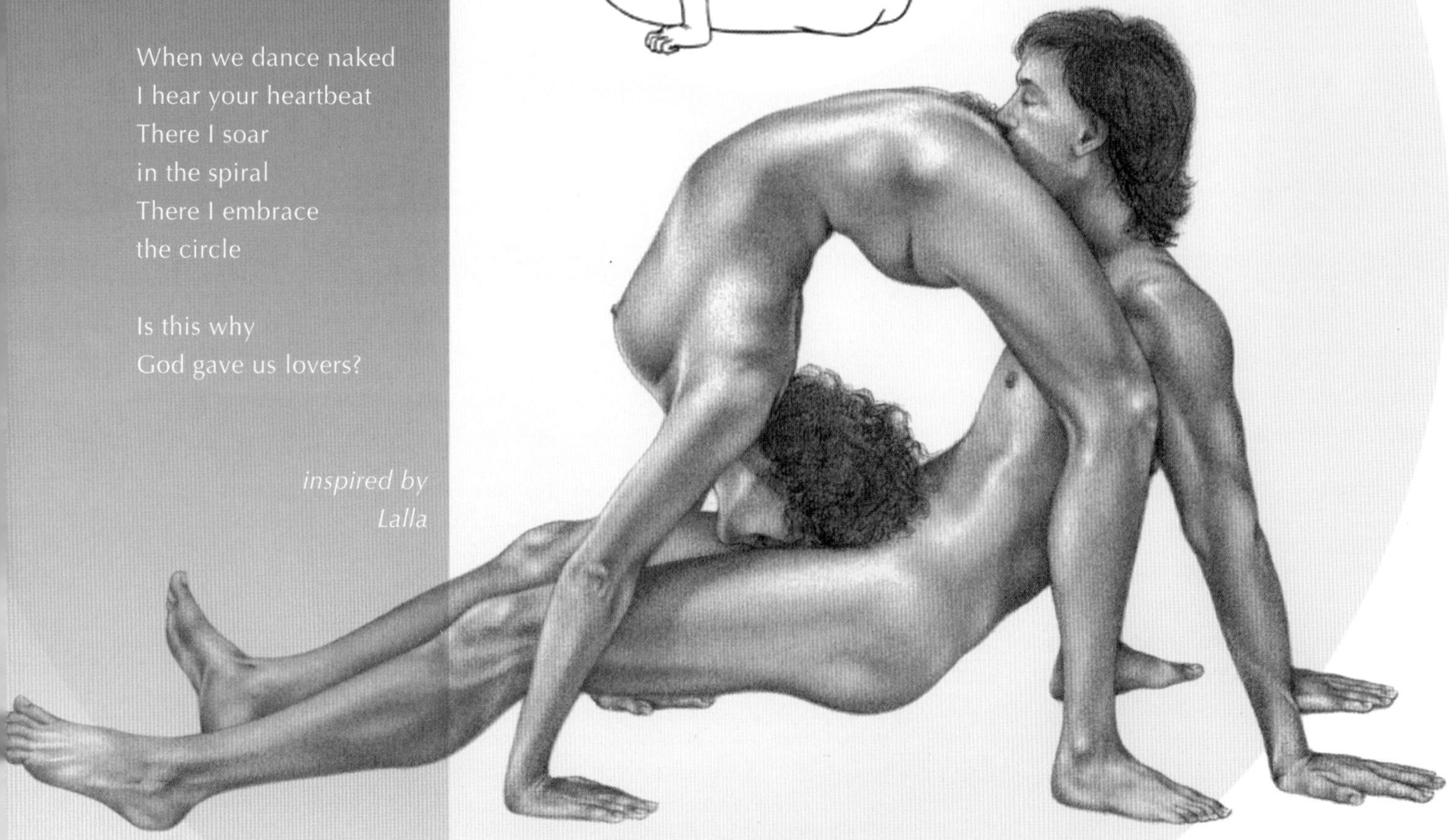

Her position should be such that her vulva is now opposite his member, the man standing up. He introduces his member and then begins to swing her, first away from him, then toward him. He thus alternately introduces and withdraws his member, and so he continues until he ejaculates.

The somersault

The woman should let her trousers fall to her ankles so that they are like fetters. She then bends down till her head is in her trousers, when the man, holding her legs, pulls her over onto her back. He then kneels down and penetrates her. It is said that there are women, who, when lying on their back, can put their feet under their head without the help of their hands or trousers.

The ostrich's tail

The woman lies on her back, and the man kneels at her feet; then he raises her legs and places them round his neck so that only her head and shoulders remain on the ground. Now he penetrates her.

Putting on the sock

The woman being on her back, the male sits between her legs and places his member between the lips of her vulva, which he grasps with the thumb and first finger. He then moves so that the part of his member which is in contact with the woman is subjected to rubbing, and continues so until her vulva is moist with the liquid which escapes from his penis. Having thus given her a foretaste of pleasure, he enters her completely.

The mutual view of the buttocks

The man lies on his back, and the woman, turning her back to him, sits on his member. He now clasps her body with his legs and she leans over until her hands touch the floor. Thus supported she has a view of his buttocks, and he of hers, and she is able to move conveniently.

Drawing the bow

The woman lies on her side, and the man, also on his side, gets between her legs so that his face is turned towards her back; now, placing his hands on her shoulders, he introduces his member. The woman then grasps the man's feet and draws them towards her; she forms thus, with the man's body, a bow to which she is the arrow.

Reciprocating motion

The man, seated on the ground, brings the soles of his feet together, at the same time lowering his thighs. The woman then sits on his feet and clasps his body with her legs and his neck with her arms. The man then grasps the woman's legs, and, moving his feet toward his body, carries the woman within reach of his member, which he introduces. By a movement of his feet he now moves her backward and forward. The woman should take care to facilitate this movement by not pressing too heavily. If the man fears that his member will be drawn right out, he must grasp the woman around the body and be satisfied with such movement as he can give with his feet.

Sitting on the member

The man sits down and stretches out his legs, and the woman sits on his thighs and crosses her legs behind his back. She places her vulva opposite his penis and lends a guiding hand. She then puts her arms around his neck, and he puts his round her waist and raises and lowers her on his member, in which movement she assists.

Coition from behind

The woman lies face downward and raises her buttocks with a cushion; the man lies on her back and introduces his member while she slips her arms through his elbows.

The sheep's posture

The woman kneels down and puts her forearms on the ground; the man kneels down behind her and slips his penis in her vulva, which she makes stand out as much as possible. His hands should be placed on her shoulders.

The camel's hump

The woman, who is standing, bends forward

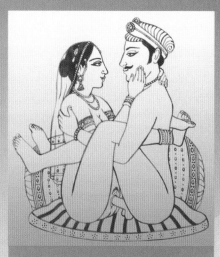

*A*re you my lover?
Or is God my lover?

Or, are you God in
human form?

My soul invokes the moon.
She whispers in the wind,
"We *all* are your lover."

I dance naked in the streets.
My tears of jubilation
      bathe my feet.

inspired by
Lalla

till her fingers touch the floor; the man gets behind and copulates, at the same time grasping her thighs. If the man withdraws while the woman is still bending down, the vagina emits a sound like the bleating of a calf, and for that reason some women object to the posture.

Standing on the wall

While facing each other, the woman, hanging with her arms round the man's neck, raises her legs and with them clasps him around the waist, resting her feet against a wall. The man now introduces his member.

The fusion of love

The woman lies on her right side and the man on his left; he stretches his bottom leg straight down and raises his other leg, letting it rest on the woman's side. Now he pulls the woman's top leg onto his body and then introduces his member. The woman may help if she likes, to make the necessary movements.

Inversion

The man lies on his back and the woman lies on him. She grasps his thighs and draws them toward her, thus bringing his member into prominence. Having guided it in, she puts her hands on the bed, one on each side of the man's buttocks. It is necessary for her feet to be raised on a cushion to allow for the slope of the penis. The woman moves. This posture may be varied by the woman sitting on her heels between the man's legs.

Riding the member

The man lies down and places a cushion under his shoulders, taking care that his buttocks remain on the floor. Thus placed, he raises his legs till his knees are close to his face. The woman then sits on his member. She does not lie down, but sits astride, as though on a saddle formed by the man's legs and chest. By bending her knees, she can now move upward and downward; or she may put her knees on the floor, in which case the man moves her with his thighs while she grasps his shoulders.

The jointer

The man and the woman sit down facing each other; the woman then puts her right thigh on the man's left thigh, and he puts his right thigh on her left one. The woman guides his member into her vagina and grasps the man's arms while he grasps hers. They now indulge in a seesaw motion, leaning backward and forward alternately, taking care that their movements are well-timed.

The stay-at-home

The woman lies on her back, and the man, with cushions under his hands, lies on her. When the introduction has taken place, the woman raises her buttocks as far as possible from the bed, and the man accompanies her in the movement, taking care that his member is not withdrawn. The woman then drops her buttocks with short sharp jerks, and, although the two are not clasped together, the man should keep quite close to the woman. They continue this movement, but it is necessary that the man be light and the bed soft; otherwise, pain will be caused.

The blacksmith's posture

The woman lies on her back with a cushion under her buttocks. She now draws her knees onto her chest so that her vulva stands out like a sieve; she then guides in the member. The man now performs for a moment or two the conventional movements. He then withdraws his member and slips it between the women's thighs in imitation of the blacksmith who draws the hot iron from the fire and plunges it into cold water.

The seductive posture

The woman lies on her back and the man crouches between her legs, which he then puts under his arms or on his shoulders. He may hold her by the waist or the arms.

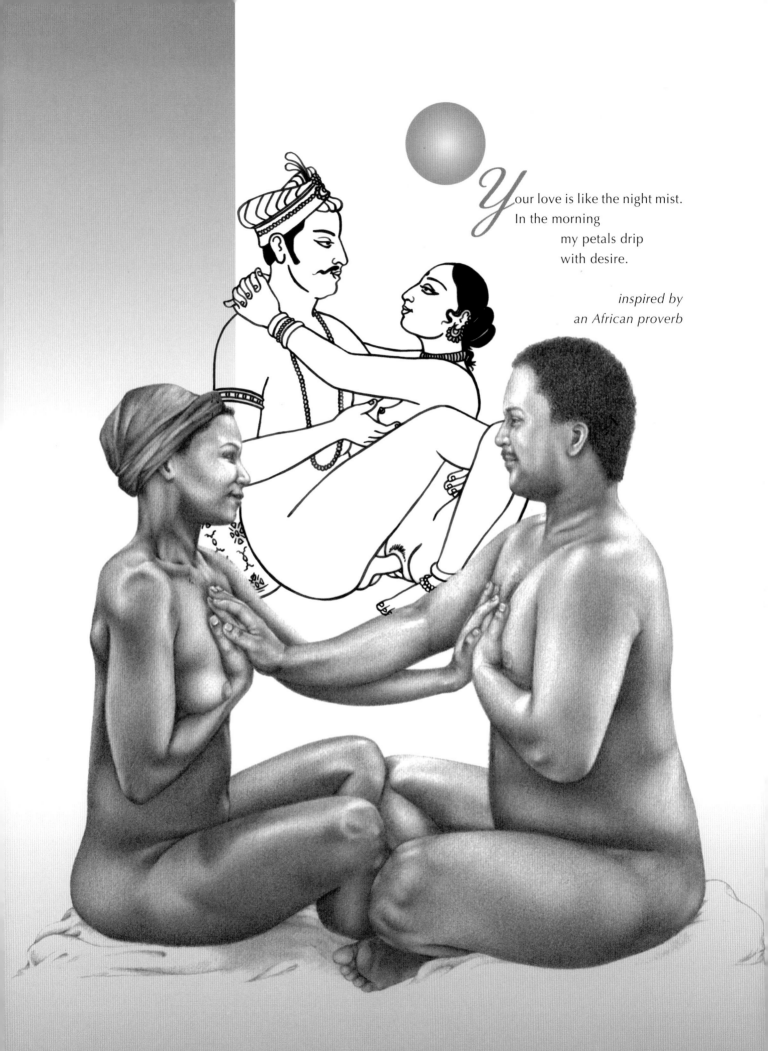

Your love is like the night mist.
In the morning
my petals drip
with desire.

*inspired by
an African proverb*

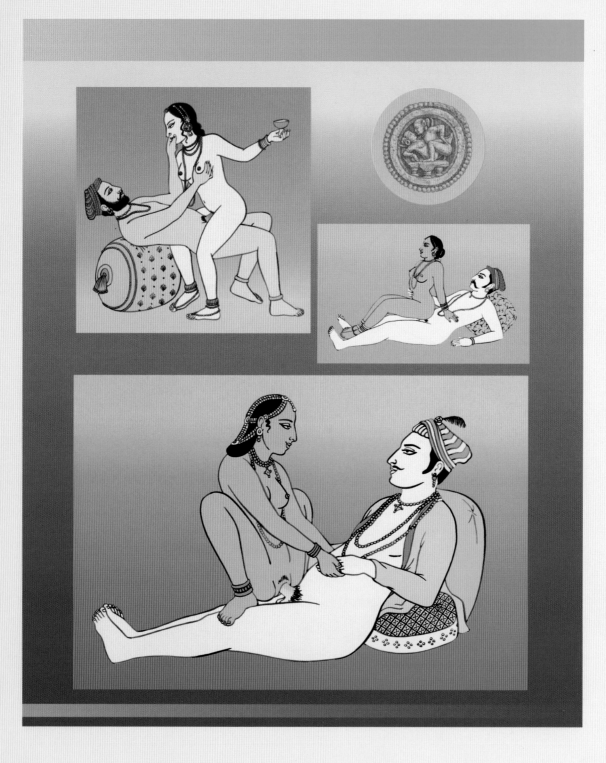

Ananga-Ranga

by
Kalyana Malla

Selected and Adapted Positions

The use of Sir Richard Burton's original translation of *husband* and *wife* remains, though most descriptions indicating the male being in charge of all the actions are edited so that the female is now more of an equal participant and initiator.

Samapada-uttana-bandha

With the wife upon her back, both legs raised and placed upon his shoulders, the husband sits close to her and enjoys her.

Nagara-uttana-bandha

With the wife upon her back, the husband sits between her legs, raises them both, keeping them on the other side of his waist, and enjoys her.

Traivikrama-uttana-bandha

When one of the wife's legs is left lying upon the bed or carpet, the other being placed upon the head of the husband, who supports himself upon both hands.

Vyomapada-uttana-bandha

When the wife, lying upon her back, raises with her hands both legs, drawing them as far back as her hair; the husband then sitting close to her, places both hands upon her breasts and enjoys her.

Smarachakrasana or the Kama's wheel position

A mode very much enjoyed by the voluptuary. In this form the husband sits between the legs of his wife, extends his arms on both sides of her as far as he can, and thus enjoys her.

Avidarita

When the wife raises both her legs, so that they may touch the bosom of her husband, who, sitting between her thighs, embraces and enjoys her.

Saumya-bandha

Given by the old poets to a form of congress much in vogue among the artful students of the Kama Shastra (ancient Vedic texts concerning sensual pleasure, which predate the Kama Sutra). The wife lies supine, and the husband, as usual, sits; he places both hands under her back, closely embracing her, which she returns by tightly grasping his neck.

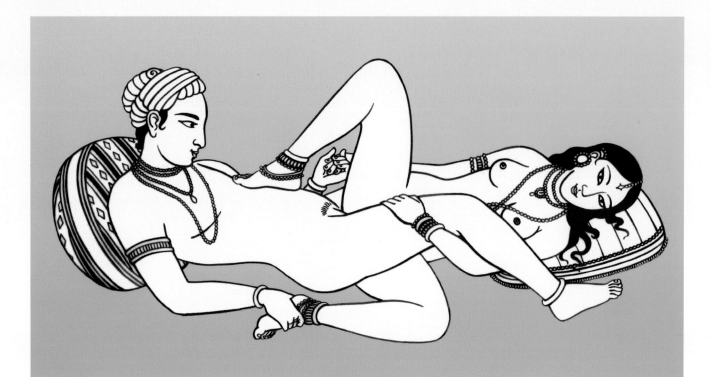

Your neck adorned with bells
        your hair braided with shells
Dance my dream awake, my love

The spring rains
        have swollen my rivers
To the beat of my drum,
        dance, dance deep into the night

inspired by the Song of Songs

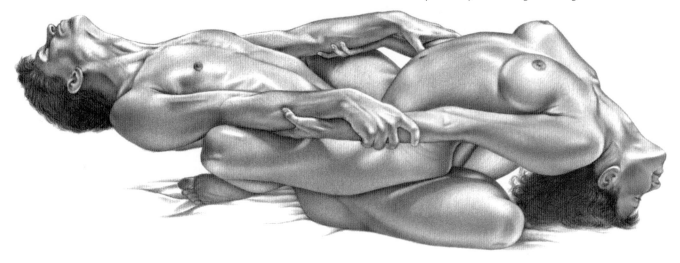

Jrimbhits-asana

The wife's body is in the form of a bow with little pillows or pads beneath her hips and head. The husband then raises the seat of pleasure and rises to it by kneeling upon a cushion. This is an admirable form of congress, and is greatly enjoyed by both.

Veshtita-asana

When the wife lies upon her back cross-legged, and raises her feet a little; this position is very well fitted for those burning with desire.

Venuvidarita

The wife, lying upon her back, places one leg upon her husband's shoulder, and the other on the bed or carpet.

Sphutma-uttana-bandah

When the husband, after insertion and penetration, raises the legs of his wife, who still lies upon her back, and joins her thighs closely together.

Vinaka-tiryak-bandha

When the husband, placing himself alongside of his wife, raises one of his legs over her hip and leaves the other lying upon the bed or carpet.

Samputa-tiryak-bandha

When both man and woman lie straight upon their sides, without any movement or change in the position of their limbs.

Karkata-tiryak-bandha

When both being upon their sides, the husband lies between his wife's thighs, one under him, and the other being thrown over his flank, a little below the breast.

Padm-asana

The husband in this favorite position sits cross-legged upon the bed or carpet, and takes his wife upon his lap, placing his hands upon her shoulders.

Upapad-asana

While both are sitting, the woman slightly raises one leg by placing her hand under it, and the husband enjoys her.

Vaidurit-asana

The husband embraces his wife's neck very closely, and she does the same to him.

Phanipash-asana

The husband holds his wife's feet, and the wife those of her husband.

Sanyaman-asana

The husband passes both the legs of his wife under his arms at the elbow, and holds her neck with his hands.

Yugmapad-asana

Is a name given by the poets to that position in which the husband sits with his legs wide apart, and, after insertion and penetration, presses the thighs of his wife together.

Vinarditasana

A form possible only to a very strong man with a very light woman; he raises her by passing both her legs over his arms at the elbow, and moves her about from left to right, but not backwards or forwards, till the supreme moment arrives.

Markatasana

Is the same position as Vinarditasana; in this, however the husband moves the wife in a straight line away from his face, that is, backwards and forwards, but not from side to side.

Knee and elbow standing-form

A posture which also requires great bodily strength in the man. Both stand opposite to each other, and the husband passes his two arms under his wife's knees, supporting her upon the inner elbows; he then raises her as high as his waist, and enjoys her, whilst she must clasp his neck with both her hands.

Hari-vikrama-utthita-bandha

The husband raises only one leg of his wife, who with the other stands upon the ground.

Kirti-utthita-bandha

This requires strength in the man. The wife, clasping her hands and placing her legs round her husband's waist, hangs, as it were, to him, whilst he supports her by placing his forearms under her hips.

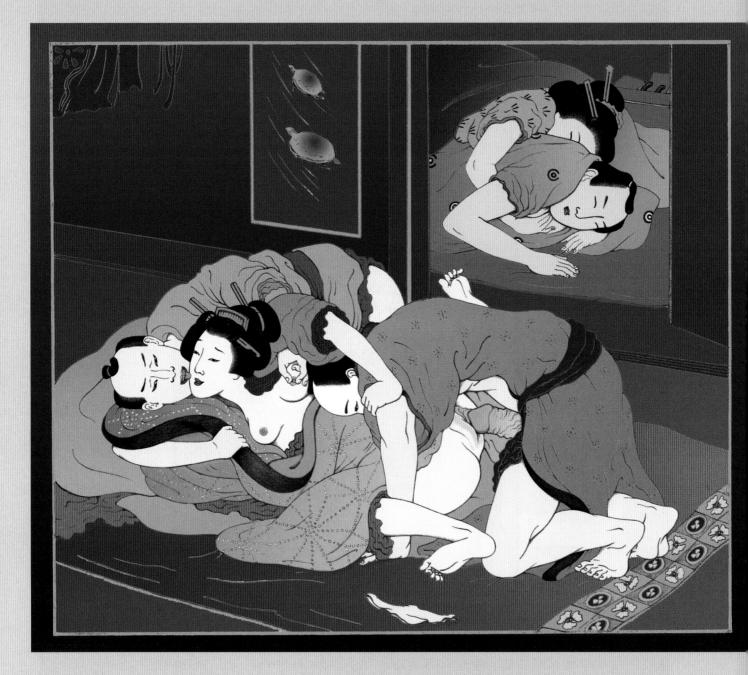

Ishimpo

by
Tamba Yasuyori

Selected and Adapted Positions

These descriptions are loose adaptations from the *Ishimpo* translation in *The Tao of Sex* by Howard S. Levy and Akira Ishihara.

The dragon turns over

With the female lying down on her back, the male lies on top of her with his thighs pressing on the mat, the female raises her vagina to receive the jade stalk, he moves about leisurely, eight shallow followed by two deep, and repeating.

The tiger's tread

The female faced downward in a crawling position, her buttocks up and head down, the male kneels behind her and embraces her belly. Then he inserts his jade stalk and penetrates deeply.

The monkey springs

The male is kneeling, and the female lies on her back with her thighs on his shoulders. Her buttocks and lower back are raised.

Cicada affixed

With the female lying front downward, the male kneels behind and inserts his jade stalk deeply into her vagina.

The tortoise mounts

The female lies on her back with her knees bent to her chest. While pushing her feet towards her breasts, the male inserts his jade stalk deeply and follows with both deep and shallow strokes.

The phoenix flutters

The female lies on her back with her knees bent and thighs pointing upward. The male crawls between her thighs and deeply inserts his jade stalk.

A rabbit sucking a hair

The male lies flat on his back, extending his legs. Facing his feet, the female straddles him, her knees to the outside.

Fish with scales joined

The male lies on his back, extending his legs. Facing his head, the female straddles him, her knees to the outside. The female moves so as to prolong her pleasure.

*The winter rains are over, my love
the rivers run swiftly*

*Come, come to my garden
and drink of my fountain*

*inspired by
the Song of Songs*

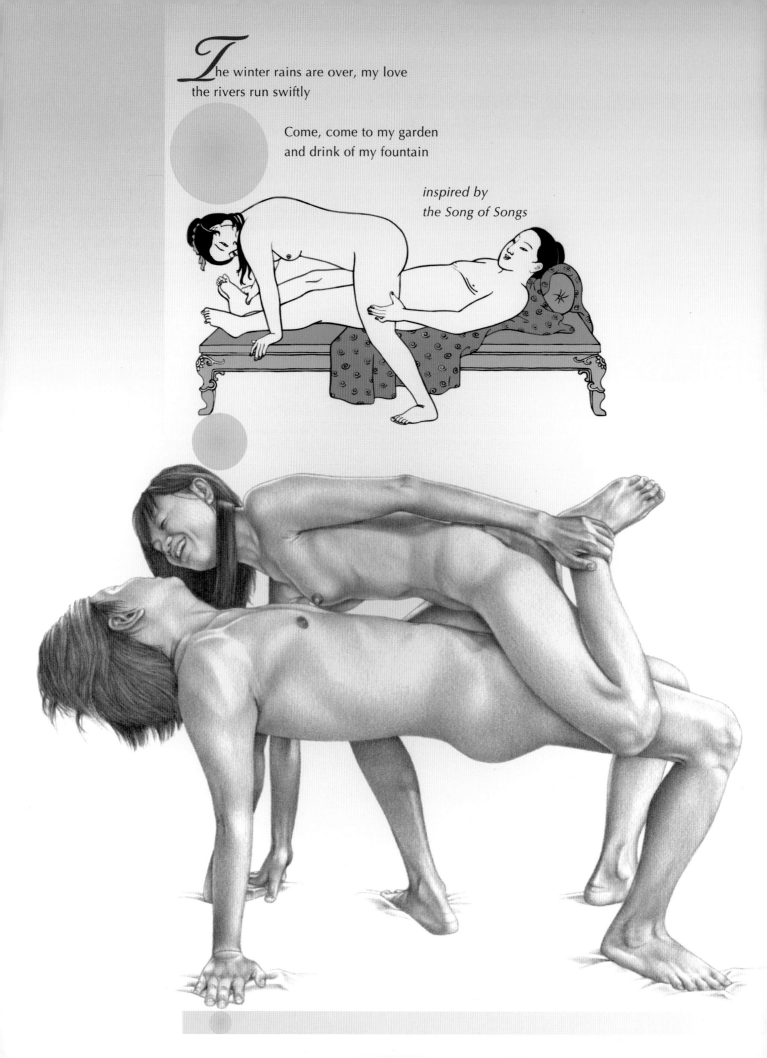

Cranes with necks intertwined

The male sits in a squatting position with the female facing him and straddling his thighs, she embraces his neck while he embraces her buttocks and assists her hip movements.

Silkworm reeling silk

The female is on her back and after the male inserts the jade stalk, she entwines both legs around his back and embraces the man's neck.

Shifting-turning dragon

The female lies on her back with both legs bent up, the male kneels at the female's thighs and with his left hand pushes both of her ankles upward and forward. He then inserts the jade stalk into the jade gate with his right hand.

Fish eye to eye

The male and the female lie down on their side face-to-face, and the female places one leg over the man. They suck each other's mouths and sip each other's tongues.

Sky-soaring butterfly

The man is on his back with both legs extended, and the female squats on top of him face to face. Then she advances with her hands his male tip into the jade gate.

The seagull soars

Standing beside the bed, the male lifts the female's legs onto his shoulders and inserts his jade stalk. Depending on the height of the bed, the female's upper back or neck and shoulders rest on the bed.

The horse's shaking hooves

The female is lying on her back, and the male lifts one of her legs onto his shoulder and inserts his jade stalk deeply.

Mountain goat facing a tree

The male sits with his legs extended, and the female straddles his thighs, facing his feet. The female then lowers her head and observes the insertion of the jade stalk while the male embraces her waist.

The donkey of early, mid, and late spring

Standing, the female bends forward, resting her hands on the bed or floor. The male stands behind, holding her waist with his hands, and inserts the jade stalk into the jade gate.

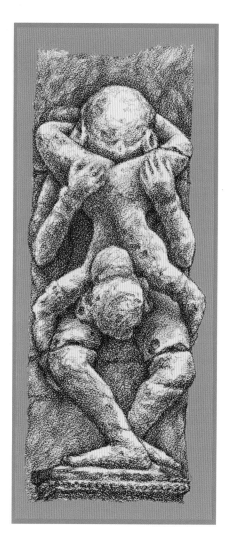

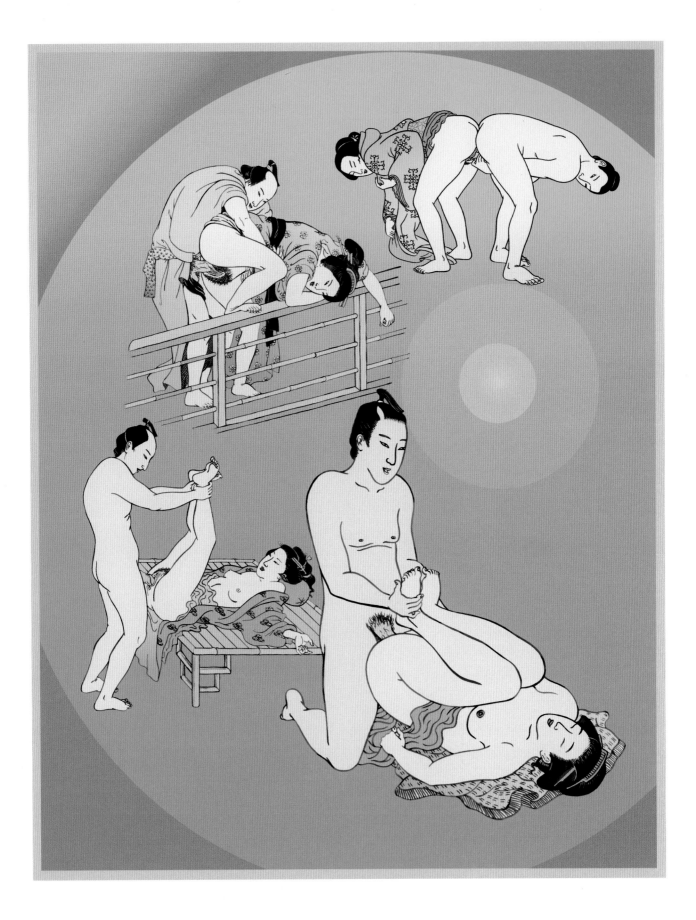

When we revel in our love's passion
through the night, I sleep not.
When you are in flight away from my lips
in the night, neither can my head find solace.

Either way,
drinking from this cup of desire, I shall die.

I pray it be in your arms.

inspired by
Rumi

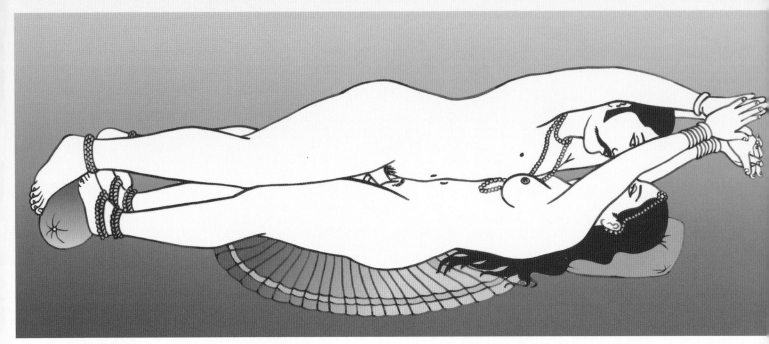

*W*here might I learn to make love?
Where might I discover my poem?

The wings of the night whisper I should seek you here in my chest.
I unlock its gate and find your flame
to light my path.

The locks of your hair reveal
you beneath.

My poem is on
your breath.

inspired by Rumi

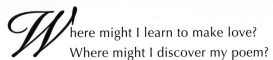

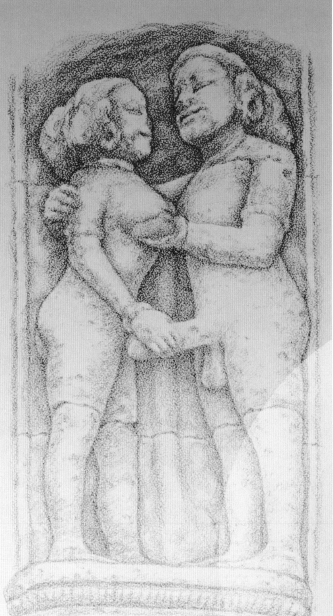

I worship at your altar
of wildflowers from the hills,
of narcissus and
apricot blossoms.
Where do you hide them,
for my vision
perceives only you?

Beloved,
when you enter my chamber,
my lips blossom into nectar,
my belly births fragrance.

Why do you wait so long
to return?

inspired by
the Song of Songs

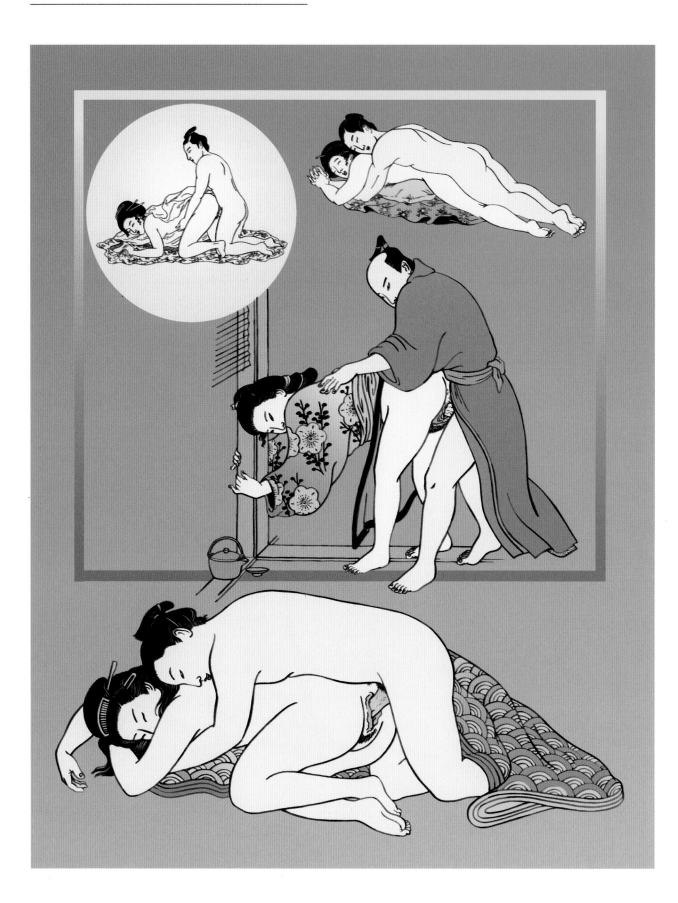

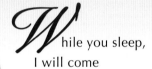

*W*hile you sleep,
I will come
    to gather spices in your garden
I will taste
    your wild honey
I will bathe in your spring stream
I will sing softly to the night
    that you might dream of love

inspired by
the Song of Songs

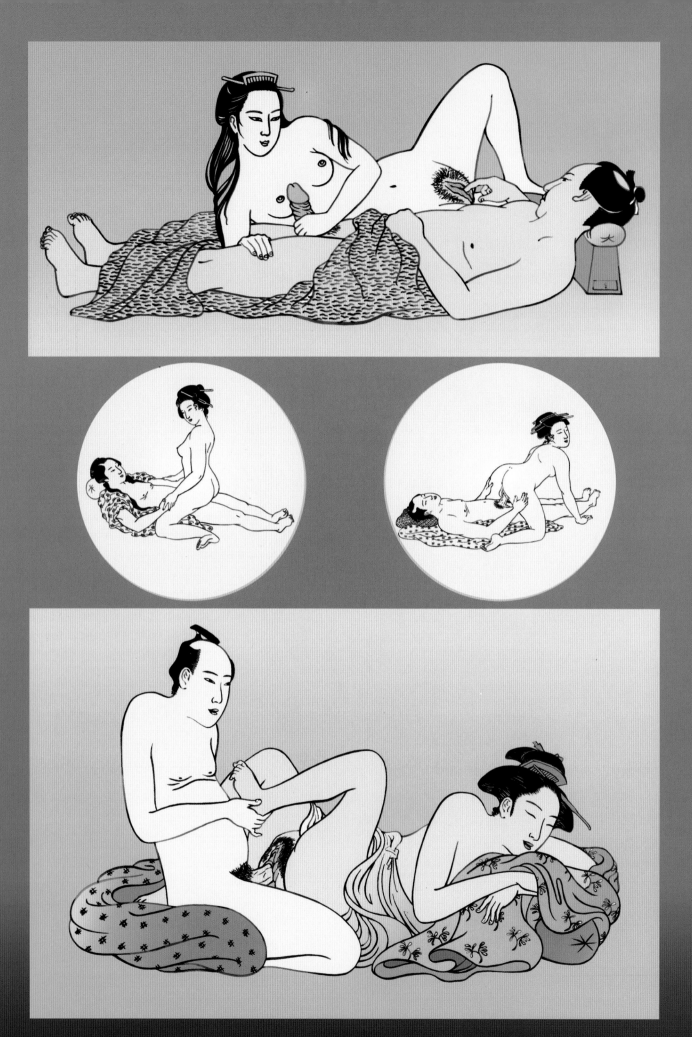

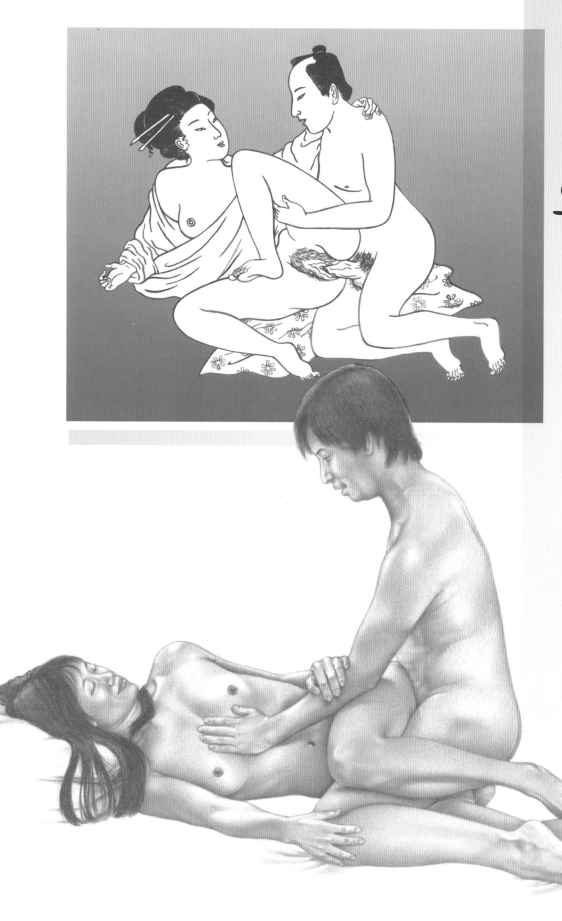

*B*eloved, you are
a secret garden
enclosed within your soul.
Where is the key
so I might drink from
your fountain?

*Beloved, the key
    is in your eyes.*

See, the door is open.

*inspired by
the Song of Songs*

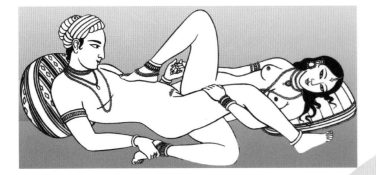

*S*ince you are but an illusion
singing my songs in my day dreams,
dancing in my night dreams,

perfect in your illumination,
your soul neither seeks me
nor rejects me.

Together we burst out in one laughter
in the belly of God.

*inspired by
Longchenpa*

The wheel of love —
shall we turn it?
In the night, we know
not where it might go.

Where but through the journey
into the night, my love,
will we find the light?

inspired by
the Kama Sutra

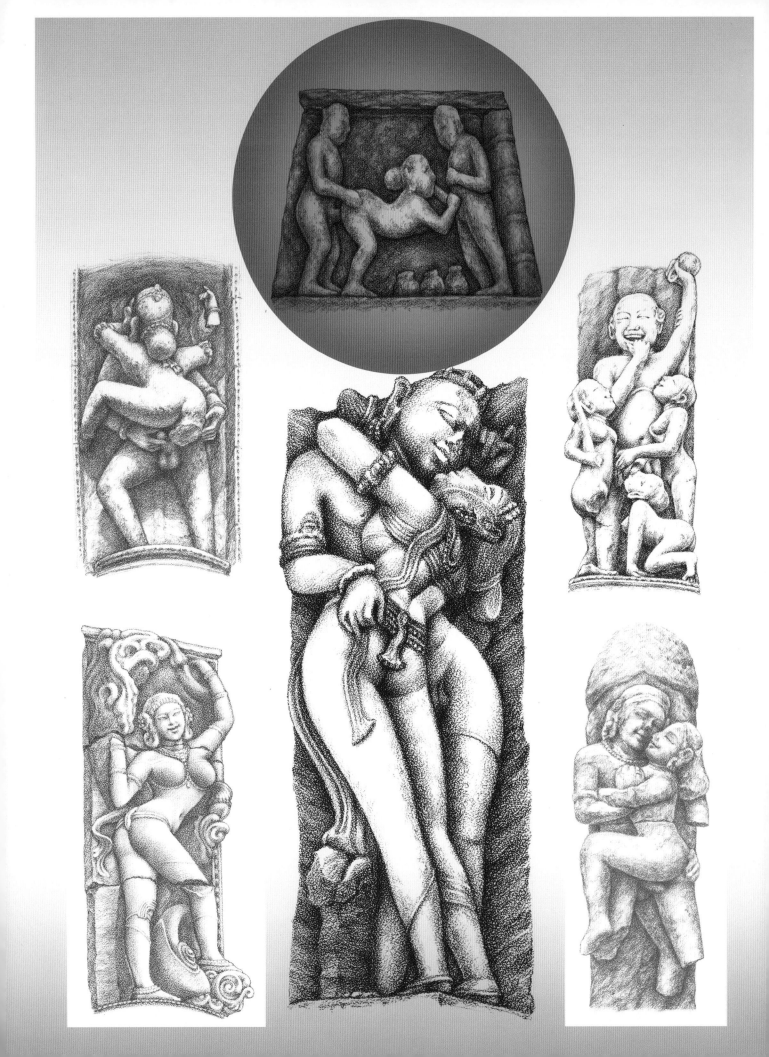

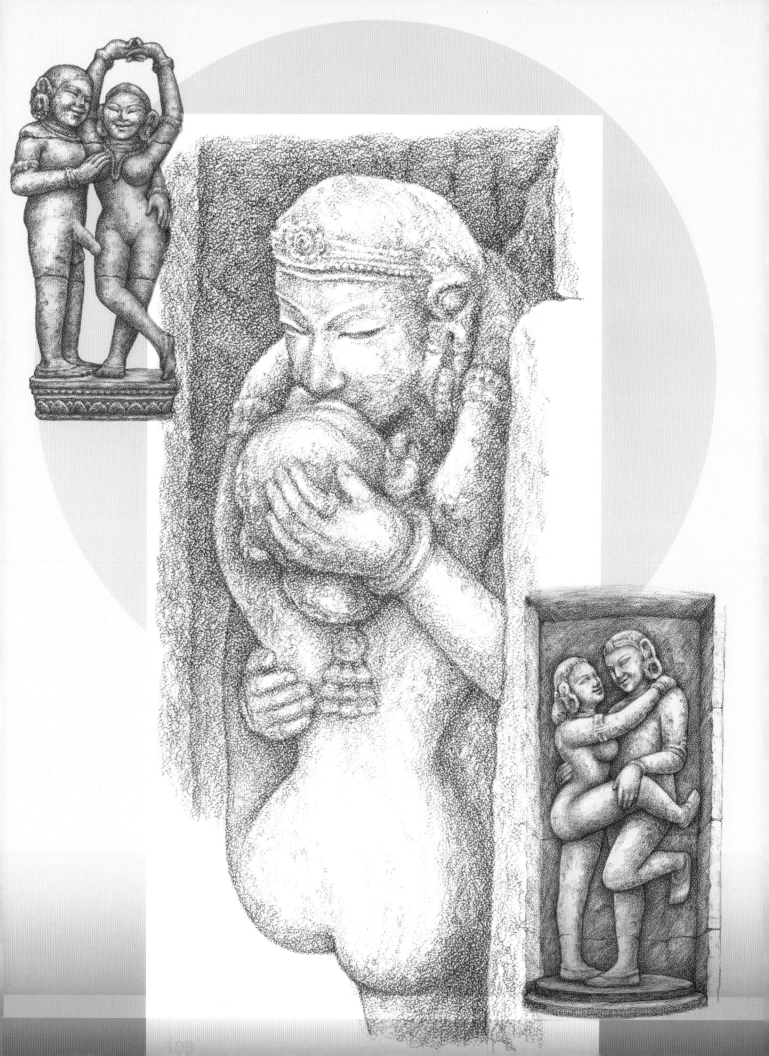

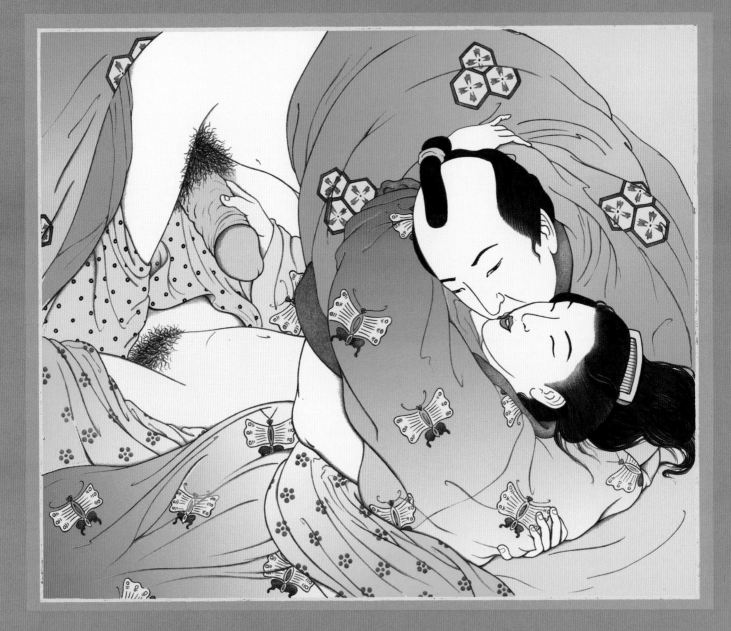

A Chronology of Sexual Embrace

- B.C.E.   means Before Common Era and is equivalent to B.C.
- C.E.   means Common Era and is equivalent to A.D.

c. 3500 B.C.E.   Possible beginning of Inanna legend in Sumer area.

c. 2700 B.C.E.   Possible birth time of the probably mythical Chinese Yellow Emperor, to whom much of the information in the Chinese sex manuals as well as the Japanese *Ishimpo* is often attributed.

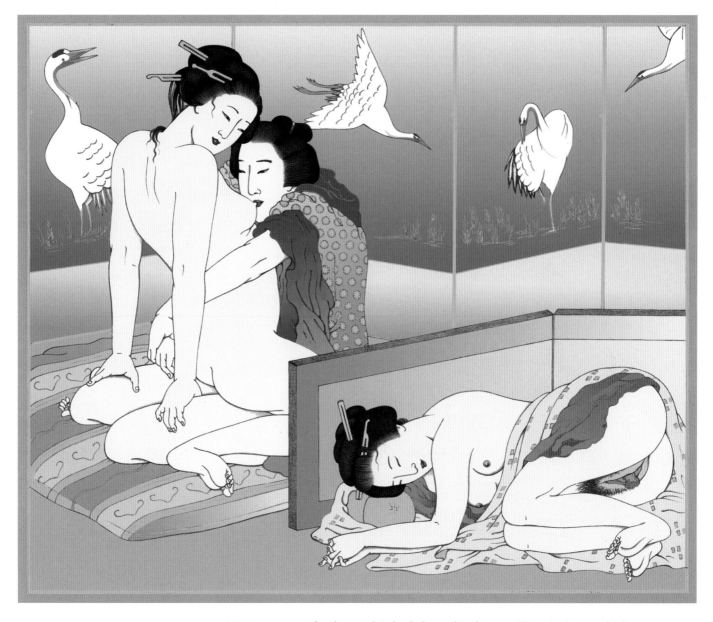

c. 2000 B.C.E.   Abraham's birth; father of Judaism, Christianity, and Islam. Born in Sumer area.

c. 1750 B.C.E.	Inanna legend written down on cuneiform tablets in Sumer.
c. 1050 B.C.E.	Solomon reigns over an empire and a harem of possibly up to 700 wives and 300 concubines. Possibly writes the biblical Song of Songs.
c. 800 B.C.E.	In India, Shvetaketu summarizes the "rules of love," which are later distilled and compiled, eventually becoming the Kama Sutra.

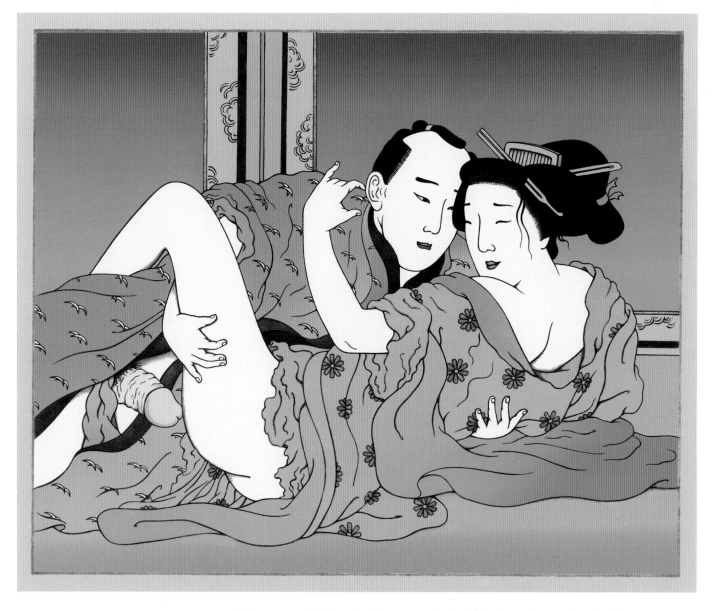

| c. 563 B.C.E. | Siddhartha Gautama, the Buddha, born in northern India. |
| c. 400–200 B.C.E. | Beginnings of Taoism as a system of philosophy in China. |

7–4 B.C.E.	Jesus born, estimated dates.
c. 200 C.E.	Beginning of Tantra movement in India.
c. 300–400 C.E.	Kama Sutra written by Vatsyayana in India, various estimated dates of writing. Alain Daniélou, in a new translation in 1994, places the writing during the fourth century C.E., with the texts from which the Kama Sutra is compiled going back to at least the third century B.C.E.,

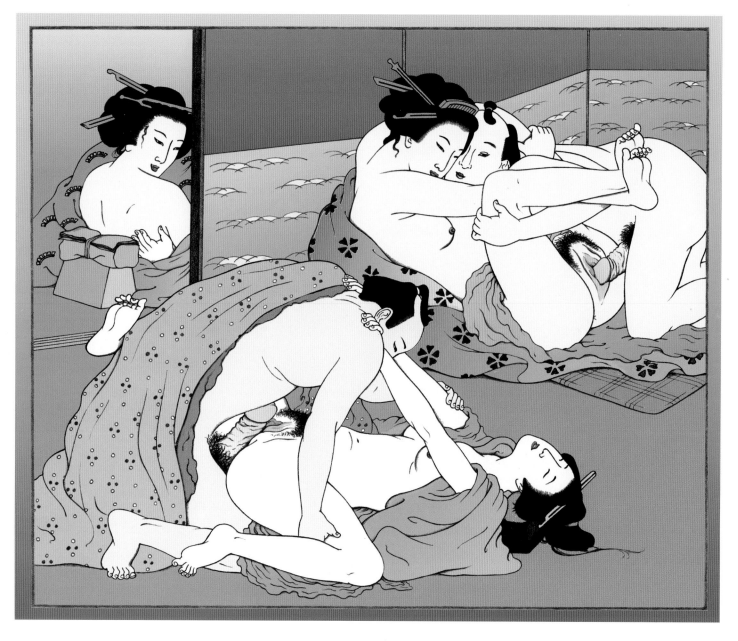

with an earlier source work coming from Shvetaketu in the eighth century B.C.E.

c. 570 C.E.   Mohammed born.

984 C.E.   *Ishimpo* written by Tamba Yasuyori in Japan: a compilation of many earlier Chinese writings with Taoist influences.

c. 1000 C.E.   Khajuraho temples built in India, with some of the world's finest erotic sculpture.

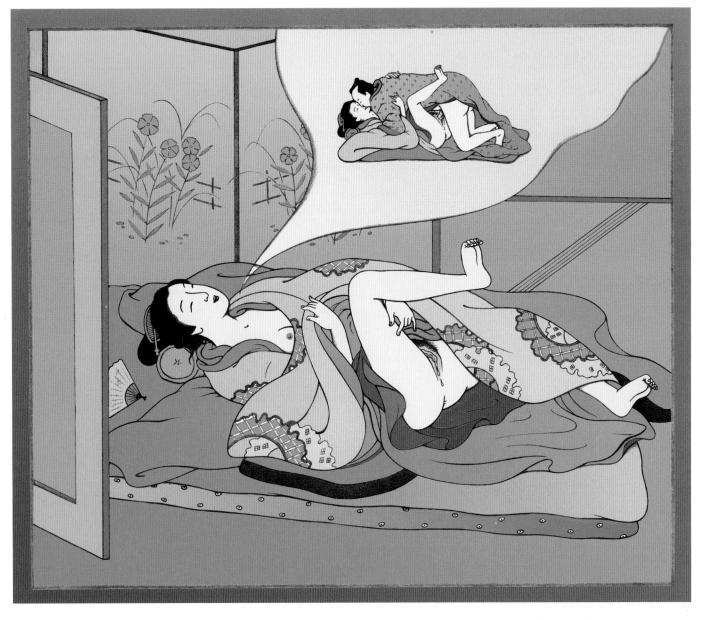

c. 1200 C.E.   *Ananga-Ranga* written by Kalyana Malla in India.

1231, 1251 C.E. Formal beginnings of the Christian Inquisitions, lasting over 500 years.

c. 1250 C.E.   Konarak temples constructed in India, displaying extensive erotic sculpture.

c. 1500 C.E.	*The Perfumed Garden* written by Sheikh Nefzawi in North Africa.
1660–1860 C.E.	Japanese shunga art style flourishes, displaying uninhibited sex.
1870 C.E.	*Ishimpo* rediscovered by the Chinese in Japan.

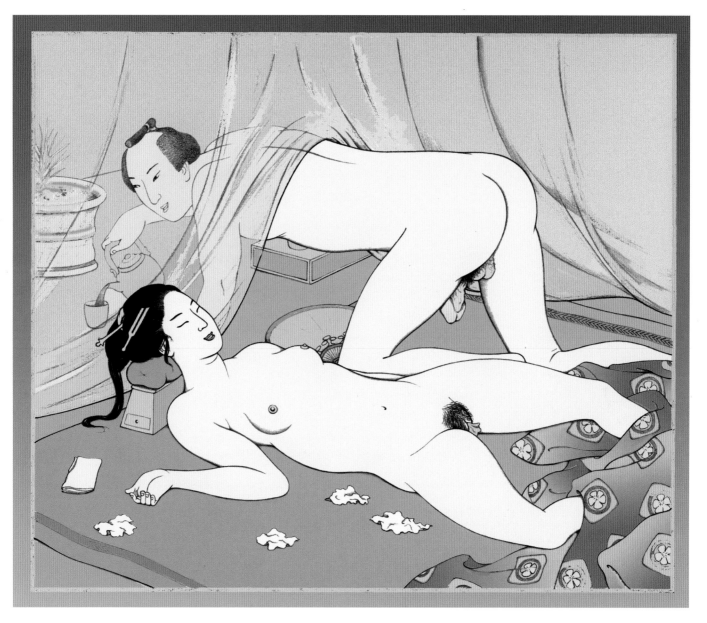

1883 C.E.	Kama Sutra translated into English.
1885 C.E.	*Ananga-Ranga* translated into English.
1886 C.E.	*The Perfumed Garden* translated into English.
1890 C.E.	Sir Richard Francis Burton dies, and his wife immediately burns most of his unpublished erotological translations and writings.

1933 C.E.	Nazis burn books and records from the prominent Institute for Sexology in Berlin.
1948 C.E.	Kinsey's *Sexual Behavior in the Human Male* published.
1953 C.E.	Kinsey's *Sexual Behavior in the Human Female* published.
1960s C.E.	Birth control pill popularized.
1966 C.E.	Masters and Johnson's *Human Sexual Response* published.

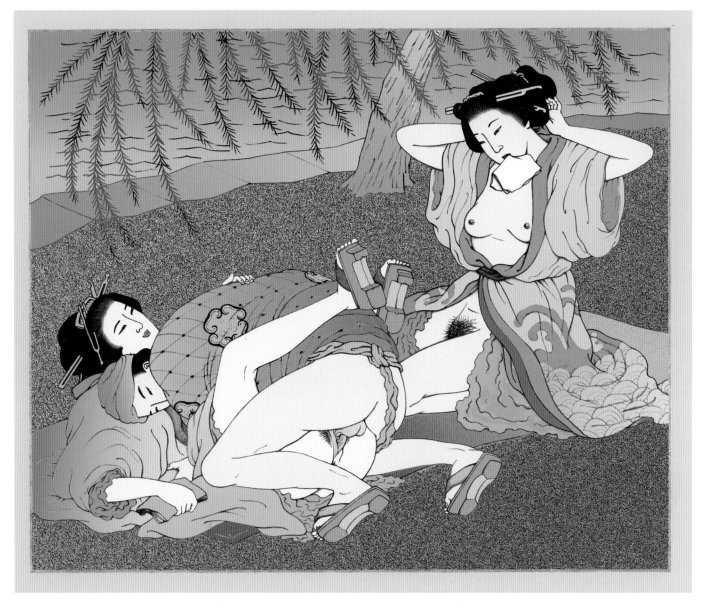

| 1968 C.E. | *Ishimpo*'s section on sexuality translated into English as *The Tao of Sex*. |
| 1970 C.E. | Masters and Johnson's *Human Sexual Inadequacy* published. |

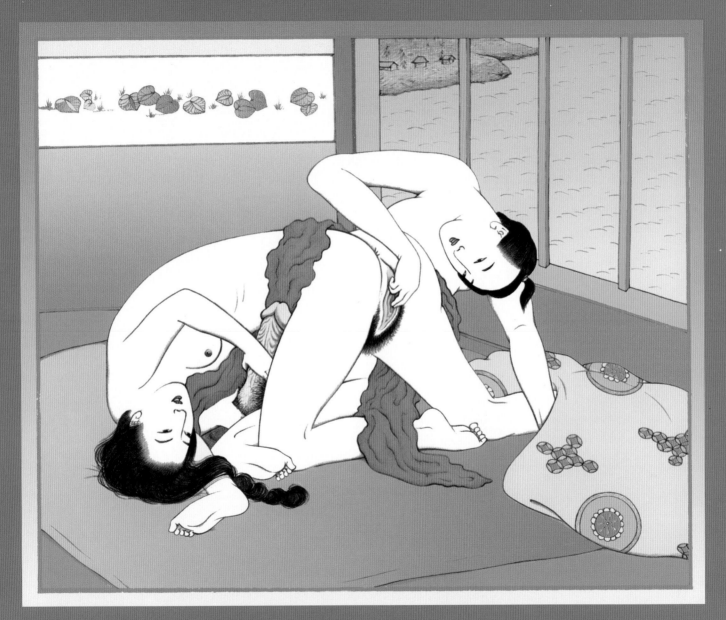

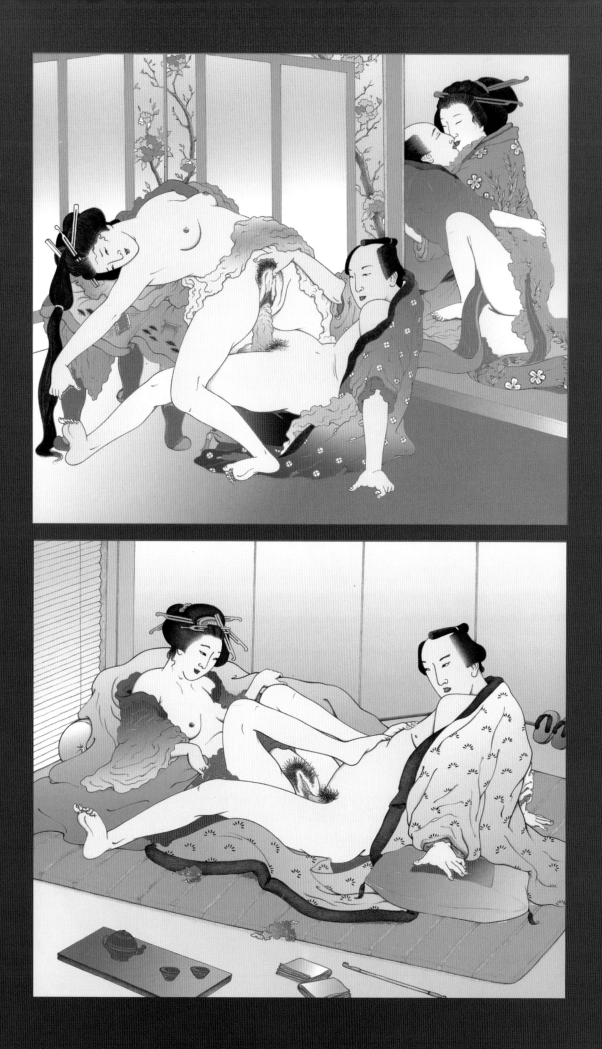

About the Author and Artists

The Author

Kenneth Ray Stubbs, Ph.D., is a certified sexologist and a certified masseur. Originally trained as a sociologist, he eventually studied and gave trainings in massage and sexuality for both the general public and sex therapists throughout North America and Europe. He has also taught as an adjunct faculty member at the Institute for the Advanced Study of Human Sexuality in San Francisco and is the author of eight books on sexuality, as presented on his website: **www.sexandspirit.com.**

The Illustrator

Kyle Spencer is a freelance illustrator residing in Oakland, California. She has a bachelor's degree from the Academy of Art College in San Francisco. Her art also appears in *Erotic Massage*, *The Essential Tantra*, *Erotic Passions*, and *Kiss of Desire*, as well as in *Tantra: The Magazine* and *Ecstasy Journal*.

The Designer

Richard Stodart has been a professional artist for more than twenty-five years. A native of Trinidad, West Indies, his images have been described as "sensitively thoughtful yet translucent, combining the wild electricity of wakefulness with the vivid languour of lucid dreaming." His works appear in magazines and as book covers and illustrations. Richard can be contacted at 512 Old Glebe Point Road, Burgess, VA 22432. For more on his work as well as purchasing information, visit his website: **www.crosslink.net/~stodart**

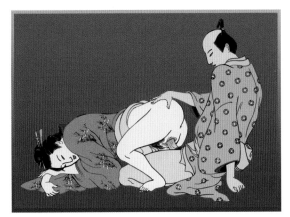

Acknowledgments

Kyle Spencer, the illustrator, indeed is able to show us the fun, the joy, and the intimacy sex can be. She brings such a soft sensuality to images of the lovers' dance. I am deeply grateful for her abilities and support. The different illustration styles here span almost a decade of her artistic development.

Richard Stodart, another accomplished artist, has creatively developed this book's cover, contributed significantly to the layout design, and colored Kyle's original black-and-white illustrations. I am honored by his friendship and artistic inspiration.

Several individuals were instrumental in advising which sexual positions to include. Harley SwiftDeer Reagan, Jwala, and Louise-Andrée Saulnier played principal roles. Also, I often gave Kyle a free hand in selecting from the myriad of photographs and illustrations from many different sources.

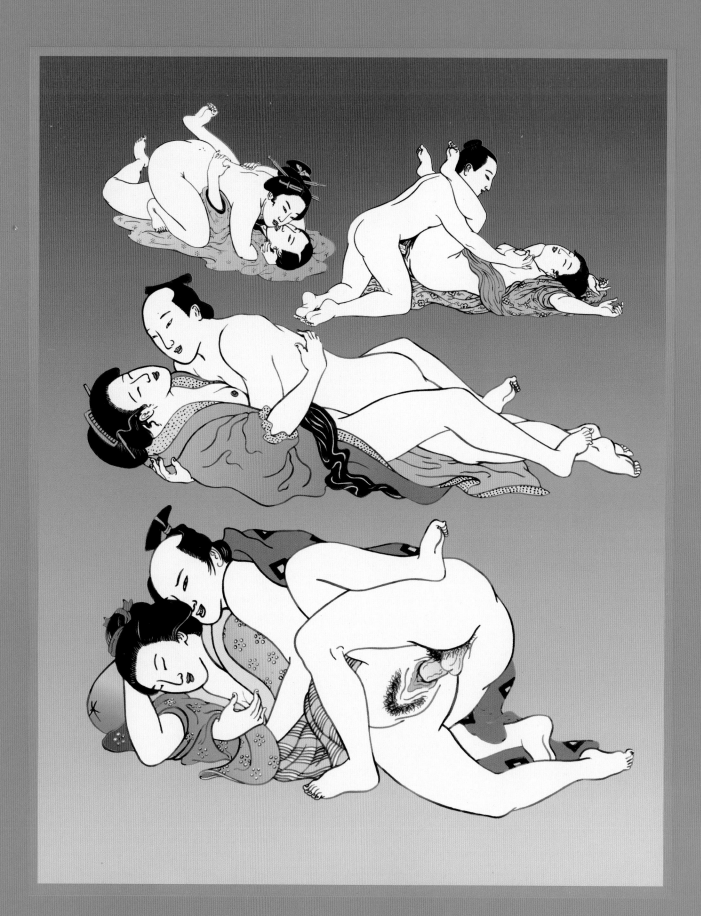